THE UNSEEN THINGS

THE UNSEEN THINGS

WOMEN, SECRECY,

HIV IN NORTHERN

NIGERIA

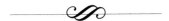

KATHRYN A. RHINE

INDIANA UNIVERSITY PRESS

Bloomington & Indianapolis

This book is a publication of

Indiana University Press
Office of Scholarly Publishing
Herman B Wells Library 350
1320 East 10th Street
Bloomington, Indiana 47405 USA

iupress.indiana.edu

♾ The paper used in this publication
meets the minimum requirements of the
American National Standard for Information Sciences—Permanence of Paper
for Printed Library Materials, ANSI
Z39.48-1992.

Manufactured in the United States of
America

Library of Congress Cataloging-in-
Publication Data

Names: Rhine, Kathryn, author.
Title: The unseen things : women, secrecy,
and HIV in northern Nigeria / Kathryn A.
Rhine.
Description: Bloomington : Indiana
University Press, 2016. | Includes
bibliographical references and index.
Identifiers: LCCN 2016001266| ISBN
9780253021311 (cloth : alk. paper) |
ISBN 9780253021434 (pbk. : alk. paper) |
ISBN 9780253021519 (ebook)
Subjects: LCSH: HIV-positive
women—Nigeria—Social
conditions. | HIV-positive
women—Behavior—Nigeria. | HIV-
positive women—Nigeria—Attitudes.
AIDS (Disease) in women—Nigeria. |
Secrecy.
Classification: LCC RC607.A26 R458
2016 | DDC 362.19697/92009669—dc23
LC record available at http://lccn.loc.gov
/2016001266

1 2 3 4 5 21 20 19 18 17 16

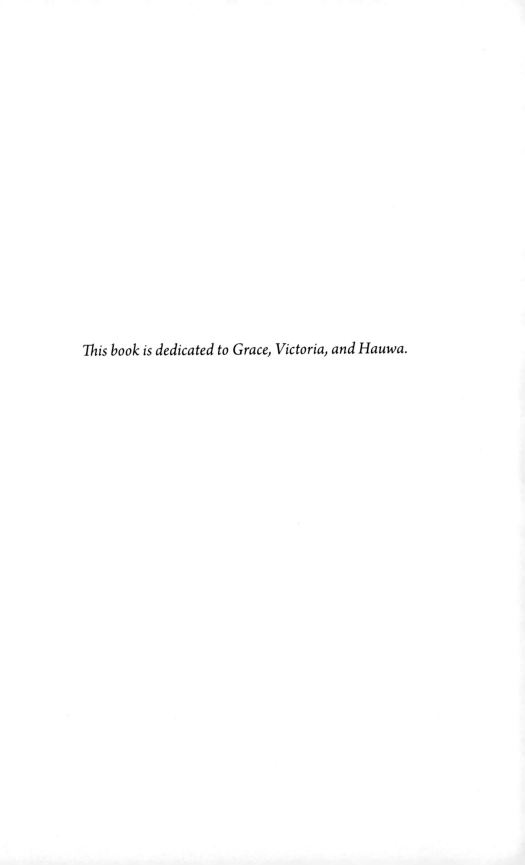

This book is dedicated to Grace, Victoria, and Hauwa.

CONTENTS

ACKNOWLEDGMENTS

THE UNSEEN THINGS first began as a research proposal I wrote as an undergraduate nearly 15 years ago. I have thus accumulated so many debts to people and institutions that it is nearly impossible to recognize them all here. Moreover, in a book about secrecy and the dignity people seek through privacy, public acknowledgements to those who have contributed the most are difficult. I am grateful to many individuals – some of whom I cannot name. The women you read about in this text, and so many more, have generously taken me into their homes and lives, devoting long hours to teaching me about their society and sharing deeply personal stories. I have been fortunate to have their companionship, patience, and trust throughout this challenging project.

My motivation for this research first came from an inspiring group of individuals at a camp for families affected by HIV in the United States. I am particularly grateful for the introduction that Lauren Wood gave me to her colleague, Samuel Adeniyi-Jones at the National Institutes of Health, who convinced me that Nigeria was an important place to learn more about antiretroviral therapies and the prevention of mother-to-child transmission of HIV. He, in turn, introduced me to Alash'le Abimaku at the Institute for Human Virology, who enthusiastically supported my plans for a year of research in Jos, Nigeria. With the support of the George Washington University Honors program, and my anthropology advisor Barbara Miller, I applied for and received a William J. Fulbright

Fellowship (IIE) to Nigeria and a Boren Fellowship for Hausa language study to carry out this work.

I first began my project in 2002 among a great team of clinicians and researchers at the Plateau State Specialist Hospital, including Comfort Daniyam and Edwina Mang. I am leaving out the name of the second clinic within which I worked in order to protect the confidentiality of some of the women in this text; however, I would like to thank Chris and Mercy, the clinic staff and volunteers, and the men and women in the support group for the kindness and generosity they extended to me. Laura (Mullen) Dobson was my closest academic friend during this period. I would never have made it through my first year without her. I also had the support of the Public Affairs Section at the US Embassy in Abuja. I thank Atim George, James Moolom, and Dehab Ghebreab, as well as their colleagues at PAS for their continued assistance and encouragement.

Once I began my graduate studies in 2003, I left Jos to explore the topics of HIV, women, and family life in the northern Nigerian city of Kano. In 2004, I was fortunate to meet Halima Ben Umar at a conference, and she invited me to spend the summer with her family. There, I benefited tremendously from her network of public health colleagues, who connected me with the support group I worked with that year. While in Kano, Khadijah Ibrahim Nuhu shared her intellectual gifts and passionate spirit with me, as my research assistant, key informant, and best friend. Her unwavering support, and insight were instrumental to my findings and overall well-being in Kano. Her husband Yaro and his wonderful family opened up their house to me and provided the emotional and practical support I needed. I have fond memories of spending time with Yaro's mother, Habiba and Bala, Maryam and Umar, Sadique and Ummi, their children, and other relatives. I equally enjoyed spending time with Khadijah's two sisters, Zainab and Rashida. I did not know it then, but Rashida would eventually make the most impact on my study, as my research assistant between 2006 and 2010. Like her sister, Rashida is fiercely smart and funny. She is a tireless, kind, and sympathetic researcher, who carefully listens and critically reflects on what she learns without reactionary judgment – a natural anthropologist.

In 2005, I spent time in both Jos and Kano to narrow my research focus. I had the great privilege of working with Kate (Bowler) Sabot while she conducted her MPH fieldwork on HIV-positive women's reproductive intentions. I also met Bola Gobir, Abdulatif Salisu, and Muyi Aina, and so many others who were charged with rolling out PEPFAR in those first few years. I am inspired by their hard work and sense of humor through it all.

The majority of the fieldwork, upon which this book is based, was conducted between 2006 and 2008 and was funded by the National Science Foundation and the US Department of Education. Over this period, with subsidized HIV testing and treatment programs underway, I worked closely with a faith-based hospital in Kano, which provides antiretroviral therapies and clinical care to over a thousand HIV-positive men, women, and children. I would like to thank Mudassar and his outstanding staff. The clinic generously provided me the space to conduct interviews with women from their support group. Although I cannot name everyone, I am grateful for the knowledge I gained from them.

At this hospital, there is one particular Treatment Support Specialist (I called her Patience in the book) who was instrumental in locating women for me to interview. I followed her in her day-to-day work, learning everything she could teach me about the marital and reproductive dilemmas faced by HIV-positive women. In addition, I often stayed in her house, ate her delicious cooking, and traveled with her to visit other patients and family in different cities across northern Nigeria. Patience is a true friend. This book would never have emerged without her.

During these years, I also conducted a survey and completed interviews with over a hundred HIV-positive women in two hospitals, as well as three additional support groups. There were numerous non-governmental organizations across Kano and Abuja, who also opened their doors to me. Dr. Yusuf Adamu helped facilitate an affiliation with the Department of Geography at Bayero University Kano, and introduced me to colleagues at the university including one of my hosts, Dr. Koguna, with whom I stayed in the old city of Chedi. In 2006, I met the Ammouri family, who quickly became some of my closest friends. I am so lucky to know Jalal, Nada, Mohamad, Maryam, Manal, and of course, Durba, who keep me thoroughly entertained and well-fed every time I travel to Nigeria.

During particularly stressful periods of fieldwork, I was fortunate to be able to fall back on my long-time friends Brent and Eugenie Friedrichs in Jos, who have so much love for the country – and always had a chair open for me on their patio at 4PM for a Star beer and peanuts. I also spent a month with Laura Arntson in Abuja, where we also became fast friends. Laura continually reminds me of the applied significance of this project and is a staunch advocate for the field of anthropology in the public health arena. I am grateful for the opportunities that USAID and the US Embassy in Abuja gave me to present my work to them.

I am indebted to Daniel J. Smith, my advisor in the Department of Anthropology at Brown University, along with the members of my committee, Marida Hollos, Pat Symonds, and Kris Peterson, my outside reader, for their careful reading and feedback. Dan's generous and committed attention, in particular, helped advance my scholarship in numerous critical dimensions. I was very fortunate to receive advice and feedback over the years from a number of other faculty members, including: Nick Townsend, Lina Fruzzetti, Phil Leis, Kay Warren, Cathy Lutz, and David Kertzer. The Population Studies & Training Center also provided me substantial support. I am especially grateful for the assistance Kelley Smith gave me.

My final year at Brown, the Cogut Center for the Humanities offered me a congenial environment for reflection and writing. A wonderful group of faculty and graduate student fellows including Sarah Moran and Sarah Wald also helped me see this project to its conclusion. I was lucky to be surrounded by many enthusiastic and empathetic students at Brown, including: Bruce Whitehouse, Salome Wawire, Brooke Bocast, Maya Judd, Andrea Maldonato, Kathleen Millar, Inna Leykin, Kristin Skrabut, Laura Varez, Jennifer Ashley, Harris Solomon, Sohini Kar, and Susan Ellison, who gave me thoughtful suggestions to my work. In 2008–2009, I received an Andrew W. Mellon Foundation/ACLS Doctoral Dissertation Completion Fellowship, which provided support for me to focus solely on writing and finish my degree.

In 2009, I joined the Department of Anthropology at the University of Kansas as an assistant professor. I received several grants to conduct fieldwork and write this book. These included a Franklin Research Grant from the American Philosophical Society and a Postdoctoral Fellowship from the West African Research Association. In addition, I received a New Faculty General Research Fund (NFGRF) grant, and research and travel support from the College of Liberal Arts & Sciences, the Kansas African Studies Center, the Office of International Programs, and the Center for Global & International Studies. I had considerable support from the Hall Center for the Humanities, including a Friends of the Hall Center book publication award, and most importantly, a faculty fellowship, which provided a semester-long teaching release in order to dedicate my time to writing. I am grateful for the help and support of Victor Bailey, Sally Utech, and especially Kathy Porsch.

Over this period, I also participated in a number of conferences, in which I met and obtained feedback from several discussants who generously read my works-in-progress. In particular, I would like to thank Adeline Masquelier, Rebecca Lester, Matthew Korhmann, Janet McGrath, Holly Wardlow, and Elisha Renne who all provided me intellectual insight and probing questions. In 2014, Jan Brunson, Megan McCullough, Karin Friederic, and Jennifer Aengst organized and edited a special issue of *Ethnos* titled, "Love and Sex in Out-of-the-Way Places," and they included my essay, "HIV, Embodied Secrets, and Intimate Labour in Nigeria." They each read and edited numerous drafts of the article. In 2015, Elisabeth McMahon and Cori Decker co-edited a special issue of *Africa Today* based on the workshop *Love and Sex in Islamic Africa*, hosted by Tulane University. They included my article, "She Lives Dangerously," and also provided substantial and helpful comments.

The participants in the 2010 conference I organized, *Medical Anthropology in Global Africa*, which led to an edited volume, pushed me to consider how my work draws from and advances decades of anthropological scholarship on health and well-being in sub-Saharan Africa. I am grateful for the experience, as well as the chance to work with and host so many Africanist scholars and friends in Lawrence.

Over 2013–2014, I was awarded a Core Fulbright Scholar Teaching & Research Fellowship (CIES) to research and teach in Lagos, Nigeria. I was hosted by the Federal Neuropsychiatric Hospital in Yaba, with the support of Dr. Rahman Lawal, the Chief Medical Director, and additional assistance from Jide Raji, Chinyere Okonkwo, Paulina Okanlawon, and several other clinicians and staff members. I was kept in good spirits at the Guest Quarters, where I met many friends while grinding through these chapters. I also received incredible support from Ed Keazor, who kept me going for months with his indomitable enthusiasm. I spent time with a vibrant group of scholars across the country, who also filled me with inspiration and encouragement: Susan Shepler, Vivian Lu, Beth Philips, Shelby Grossman, Megan Turnbull, Portia Roelofs, Rudi Gaudio, Jamaine Abidogun, and Pete Kingsley. Affiong Williams also helped me brainstorm and clarify my ideas during long commutes to and from the mainland. Chi Chi Okoye gave me an important perspective onto the intersections of love and exchange in Nigeria.

I currently have the great fortune to be part of a community of interdisciplinary Africanist scholars at the University of Kansas and I have given a number of talks at the Kansas African Studies Center. Thanks especially to: Glenn Adams, Hannah Britton, Liz MacGonagle, Garth Myers, and Ebenezer Obadare. Thanks also to the Communication Studies Colloquium; the Women, Gender, and Sexuality Studies Gender Seminar; the International Programs Faculty Seminar on Global Health; and the Hall Center's Health & Humanities and Faculty seminar, where I presented multiple chapters of this text.

In the Department of Anthropology, I would like to thank David Frayer, my first-year mentor; Sandie Gray, another unyielding advocate; Allan Hanson, Brent Metz, and Don Stull, who have all provided great advice and support; and Jane Gibson, our chair, who gave last-minute assistance to one of my chapters and steady confidence throughout the process. Carlos Nash is one of my closest friends and has provided critical advice on Chapter Three. Ivana Radovanovic read every chapter with valuable feedback. In addition, I have had many students who were always willing to lend a helping hand and ask challenging questions. In particular Marwa Ghazali has read, formatted, and copyedited the entire text. Colleen Pollock prepared and archived interview transcripts and provided critical feedback. My fall 2015 Introduction to Medical Anthropology seminar read the manuscript in its entirety and gave me very thoughtful comments.

I have two colleagues in anthropology at the University of Kansas who weathered through my writing stages – from tears of resignation to frustrating blocks, to surges of ideas and optimism, and the withering, tedious copyediting labor – with humor and patience. Akiko Takeyama and John Janzen have read every word I wrote, fundamentally shaping the text in many critical ways. This book would not be the same without their friendship, support, and careful eye. I also need to single out several colleagues, who painstakingly read draft after draft of these chapters over the past decade and have helped me in more ways than I can count. I am grateful for their analytical insight and masterful power of distraction. A number of these collegial exchanges first began as graduate school friendships: Susi Keefe, Andrea Mazzarino, Rebecca Peters, and Rebecca Galemba were there for me from the very beginning. I first met Stacey Vanderhurst as she made her initial tentative steps into fieldwork in Nigeria, and now years later, I am thrilled to have her as a colleague at the University of Kansas. We have learned so much from one another.

And finally, I owe Carmen McCain an enormous intellectual and spiritual debt. Carmen was one of the first people I met in Nigeria, before either of us had any idea about where we would go to graduate school or what we would study. Our projects and questions have now intersected in many wonderful ways. Together, we conducted interviews, learned Hausa, starred in a film, and traveled across Nigeria from Sokoto to Maiduguri. We have grappled with each other's work, sentence by sentence. My research and writing would not be the same without her. Na gode kwarai da gaske.

Sections of three of the chapters included in this book have been previously published in somewhat altered forms as journal articles. A portion of chapter three, "Dilemmas of Disclosure" was published in "She Lives Dangerously: Intimate Ethics, Grammatical Personhood, and HIV in Islamic Northern Nigeria," *Africa Today* 61 (4[2015]). Chapter four, "Intimate Ethics" is derived, in part, from an article titled, "HIV, Embodied Secrets, and Intimate Labour in Northern Nigeria," in *Ethnos: Journal of Anthropology* 79 (5[2014]) available online at: http://www.tandfonline.com/doi/abs/10.1080/00141844.2013.817458.

Excerpts of chapter five, "Hope" appeared in "Support Groups, Marriage, and the Management of Ambiguity among HIV-Positive Women in Northern Nigeria," *Anthropological Quarterly* 23 (2[2009]). I am grateful to Kwame Dawes and Peepal Tree Press for their permission to reprint excerpts from the poem "Faith" from Dawes' outstanding book *Hope's*

Hospice and Other Poems (2009). Finally I would like to thank Glenna Gordon for her permission to reprint her magnificent photograph as the cover of this book.

At Indiana University Press, I would like to thank Dee Mortensen and Sarah Jacobi, as well as Ellen Foley and an additional anonymous reviewer, for their critical feedback and effort to bring this book into being.

In Lawrence, Sarah Gross, my forever roommate and now KU colleague, read the entire book with a discerning eye. My friends, Steve and Xiaowen, Tamara, Carla, Andrea, and especially Tarang Jain, were there for me every step of the way through this grueling journey.

Finally, in a book that is fundamentally about the human needs and hopes for kin, I would like to acknowledge my own family: my parents, Rose and Dave Rhine, along with Patrick, Shawn, Andy, Erin, and Nora.

THE UNSEEN THINGS

Introduction: Things Unseen

2. The Unseen Things

Hope is in the tender hands that hold you.
Hope is in the embrace of the loving.
Hope is in the flesh touching flesh
to remind us of our human selves.
Hope is in the gentle nod of recognition,
hope is in the limping body still pushing
against the pain, the discomfort, still
laughing from so deep down it feels
like the rush of alcohol in the head
the full abandonment of all fear.
Hope is in the freedom to say
I long to be touched by a lover,
I long to feel the rush of desire
satisfied; hope is to embrace hunger
and find comfort in the sharing of needs.
Hope is in the hands we grasp,
the prayers we whisper,
the Amen, the Amen, the Amen.
Kwame Dawes, *Faith*

IN THE SPRING of 2003, I met with a young, widowed woman named Mary in an HIV clinic in the middle-belt city of Jos, Nigeria.[1] It was a difficult interview, filled with many tearful pauses as she recounted her relationship history. Apart from the physicians and counselors in the hospital, I was the only person who knew she was infected with HIV. Mary's narrative jumped back and forth in time. It was hard to understand. She was anxious and interrupted at numerous points to ask questions: about America, about her health, about the tape recorder. As Mary grew comfortable with me, more personal questions followed: Did I have a boyfriend? When would I marry? I stammered through my answers. Yet another interruption: "Katie," she said, "I want your advice." Mary paused. She then asked, "Can I get married?" I did not know what to say.

Like most of the hospital staff at that time, I assumed remarriage was not an option for women like Mary. Many people told me unsettling stories of women abandoned by their families, friends, and partners when they disclosed their status. Because of this, Mary had yet to tell anyone. She continued: her doctor warned her about spreading the virus. Her pastor encouraged HIV-positive couples to marry in their church, but she was afraid to tell him about her diagnosis. Mary's family repeatedly asked about her boyfriends and introduced her to admirers, hopeful that she would remarry soon. Mary told me that she was in love and had a boyfriend. I wanted to know more, but our interview ended abruptly when she had to leave.

I soon learned that many of the HIV-positive women I met worried about marriage. They actively sought out and were pursued by men interested in relationships. Women wondered: Where do you meet HIV-positive boyfriends? Must they also have HIV? Will they desert you if they learn your status? Will they tell others? Can HIV-infected couples have healthy babies? As the poet Kwame Dawes (2008) describes, even as men and women endure the emotional and physical pains of life with HIV, humans everywhere share these same dilemmas and desires: to be lovingly embraced, to be swept away by pleasure, to abandon our deepest fears, and to find comfort when we suffer. Hope is a social, spiritual, and bodily experience.

Over the past decade, I spent close to three years conducting fieldwork in HIV treatment centers and support groups across northern and middle-belt Nigeria. When I first arrived, I expected to observe hospital wards and meeting spaces filled with thin, frail, and sickly patients. This was not, in fact, my experience at all. Instead, I would often see rows of waiting room benches lined with women dressed as if they were going to a wedding or a party. The apprehensive faces and tearful eyes that I witnessed in my interviews with women like Mary were camouflaged by conspicuous displays of beauty and well-being.

Among the Hausa-speaking Muslim women waiting to collect their medications in the northern city of Kano, I noted freshly ironed dresses made from traditional cloth with matching veils. Their makeup was modest but carefully applied. Their shoes and handbags were fashionable and neatly matched one another. I admired gold earrings, bangles, necklaces, and trendy beaded jewelry in bright colors. These accessories complemented women's dresses, shoes, and hijabs. Signs of an active social life were evident in the henna designs on their hands and feet. When a woman marries, her close female friends and family members decorate their bodies for the wedding celebration.

Christian women in the clinics were equally well-dressed. While some wore "native wear," others had on Western clothes: skinny jeans or long skirts and tight T-shirts or blouses inscribed with American or European labels. Their hair was carefully coifed, recently relaxed, braided, or tied with extensions. Women would occasionally take out a compact or a small mirror and reapply powder, eyeliner, or lip gloss, mindful of the fact that their beauty keeps them at the center of attention in the room.

As men cast their approving gazes upon them, these women employ such self-fashioning efforts to mask their status from the questioning eyes of uninfected persons. No one would suspect well-dressed, self-assured, and evidently thriving women of being HIV-positive. Their appearances also serve to conceal histories of violence and abuse, abandonment, a myriad of illnesses, overt acts of stigma, and life in poverty. An attractive and healthy body can produce desirability, virtue, and the possibility of a family, stability, and social mobility. In short, these presentations of health and beauty signify HIV-positive women's will to survive. This book documents not only the individual ambitions and the structural constraints they face but also the most taken-for-granted dimensions of everyday life – their spoken *and unspoken* statements of hope in the aftermath of an ignominious diagnosis.

In the early years of the epidemic, much of the news we heard about Africa were counts and accounts of the dead and dying. The numbers are staggering. More than 75 million people worldwide have contracted the virus and nearly 36 million have died from AIDS-related complications.[2] From the time physicians first identified HIV in the country in 1986, Nigerians have accounted for at least three million of these fatalities.

Initial responses in the country were characterized by widespread denial and gross misunderstandings. In an attempt to counter suspicions of HIV as a fictitious disease, early public health campaigns used pictures of skeletons, blood, and coffins to accompany awareness messages, such as, "AIDS kills: Protect yourself," and "If you think you can't get AIDS, you're *dead* wrong." As a result, the Hausa terms for HIV suggest an irreversible, near-death condition. *Kanjamau* refers to a lifeless body that is virtually skin and bones, and *kabari kusa* figuratively means, "one foot in the grave." These names and images reinforce the virus's fatal connotation.

Despite reports that projected a dramatic increase in HIV prevalence over the 1990s, the federal government did little to scale up its public health infrastructure.[3] Most Nigerians who contracted HIV lived with and died from a fatal illness with an unspeakable cause. Then, very few of the country's infected patients were even tested. Many of the women who learned their status during this period did so only after they witnessed the death of husbands, boyfriends, and babies. They grappled with questions such as: Why am I sick? How can I manage the pain of dying? What will I do when my husband passes away? Who will care for my children when I die? Will there ever be a cure?

I began my ethnographic research among HIV-positive women on the cusp of a major epidemiological and epistemological shift. In 2003, motivated in part by national security concerns, the United States Congress approved the President's Emergency Plan for AIDS Relief (PEPFAR) to provide free antiretroviral therapies to countries most affected by the epidemic.[4] Nigeria, with the second highest number of HIV-infected persons in the world, was among the first to be recognized by PEPFAR and receive support for its prevention, treatment, and care initiatives.

Since 2003, the number of people collecting subsidized medications in Nigeria has grown close to 500,000, with as many as 1.5 million or more under medical supervision and on waiting lists for treatment.[5] Antiretroviral therapies have transformed the illness into a manageable chronic condition. While patients have not been granted a life free of disease, a positive diagnosis no longer means a death sentence, as the terms above imply. The virus's most pronounced symptoms – severe weight loss, rashes, fatigue, and unrelenting coughs, among others – are much less likely to betray them.

As a result of these medical, infrastructural, and pharmaceutical advances, men and women are free to consider the possibility that other kinds of deaths unrelated to HIV, await them. Over and over, I heard people remark on this change: "At the time," one woman recalled, "I felt I would die. But later, I discovered that other healthy people get sick and die, and I am still alive, despite being infected by the virus. In fact, I have become healthier. I now do things an HIV-negative person cannot do."

Another person explained to me, "HIV-positive women dress beautifully because they have not lost hope. They believe they are alive until the day Allah takes their soul." As the epidemic advances through its third decade, antiretroviral therapies provide women vital resources for defying the virus's deadly prognosis; yet as a result, they encounter new questions over how to live meaningfully with this deeply stigmatized disease – a stigma that has remained largely unchanged since the advent of the epidemic.[6]

In this book, I explore the aspirations, dilemmas, and everyday lives of women participating in the world that HIV prevention and treatment campaigns have opened up to them. While global health interventions may indeed transform patients' overall health and life expectancy, scholars and activists often focus on the significance and consequences of antiretroviral therapies for the nation as a whole. They fail to fully consider the social relations that produce suffering and well-being among ordinary Nigerians. These relationships might enhance women's desire to adhere to treatment, undermine their effectiveness, or have nothing to do with them. Moreover, antiretrovirals alone cannot reconfigure the larger social and economic structures that constrain HIV-positive women from pursuing their ambitions and reconstituting their lives.

My goal is to examine the ways in which women obtain social, financial, and health care resources through their relationships. While most of the people I describe in this book eventually gained access to comprehensive HIV treatment, many remained in abject poverty. More than two-thirds of all Nigerians live on less than two US dollars a day. Few children from indigent families complete a university degree. Many of the women

I met did not finish secondary school. Some only received an elementary education. Although several had salaried positions, the majority of them did not have full-time work. Occupations in the informal economy rarely offer women consistent or sufficient income. To improve their economic circumstances, women frequently marry at young ages.[7] Nevertheless, poor women are more likely to be divorced or abandoned than those from more privileged backgrounds.

Because divorcees and widows lack the economic resources and symbolic protection that northern Nigerians believe marriage offers, they are scrutinized for possible moral transgressions or, alternatively, ignored altogether. Many non-married women know what it is like to beg for money only to be turned down and insulted by their relatives and friends. As a result, some have fallen sick and even lost children to treatable illnesses. An HIV-positive diagnosis exacerbates women's precarious economic positions, both because of increases in health care expenses and because the virus often unravels the relationships upon which they rely for support.

Governmental and nongovernmental agencies widely recognize the tolls poverty takes on women's health and well-being, and routinely carry out economic empowerment initiatives to address these pervasive trends. These programs have had limited success, in part because few stakeholders are aware of how and why women's relationships feature so prominently into these needs. With few material assets, Nigerians invest much of their energy, time, and money into upholding their reputations. Intimate partnerships with respectable, supportive men commonly elevate women's social status.

In political, medical, and popular discussions about the epidemic, however, there are almost no mentions of HIV-infected women's ability to feel desire, pleasure, and love. Neither scholars nor public health professionals are particularly concerned with women's efforts to provide these bodily, emotional, and social resources to others. Women thus face a difficult dilemma: How do they make claims for intimacy in their relationships while living with an invisible, yet highly stigmatized, disease? In navigating this new ethical frontier, women strive, first and foremost, to keep their status a secret from others.

The sociologist Georg Simmel (1950) writes, "The secret offers . . . the possibility of a second world alongside the manifest world; and the latter is decisively influenced by the former."[8] HIV-positive women's beauty, desirability, and health offer them the possibility of a world in which they embody normalcy, while their virus is relegated to a second, unseen world. This book argues secrets are not simply the private things, ideas, or lived experiences that escape recognition from others. Instead, they constitute a set of practices that involve actively withholding some things while emphasizing others. Secrets are situationally defined, as well as exchanged, exposed, and protected by women and their families, communities, and even health care providers. Moreover, a woman's HIV status is only one of many secrets she possesses.

In Nigeria, political and religious leaders frequently accuse young women of being greedy and promiscuous. Some suggest that they deserve HIV as punishment for these moral deficits. HIV-infected women thus not only struggle to keep their status out of public view but also attempt to conceal their sexual partnerships. In addition, as members of a society that firmly believes kinship protects a person's well-being, women often hide the fact that their husbands are unsupportive, unfaithful, and sometimes violent toward their children and them. To defend their respectability, these women may suppress their feelings of love, pleasure, and desire, as well as their disappointments, frustrations, and fears. While counselors widely promote disclosure as a fundamental part of the therapeutic process, this book aims to understand the role of discretion in HIV-positive women's pursuit of dignity.

In addressing this question, I contribute to three overlapping bodies of anthropological scholarship. First, I examine marriage and the virus's effects on the ways intimate relationships are forged and fractured in northern Nigeria. Second, I focus on women's efforts to conceal and reveal their secrets, emphasizing secrecy's performative qualities. And third, I relate these ethical acts to the labor of caregiving: practices at the core of the hopes women possess and the burdens they carry as they negotiate life with HIV in the era of antiretroviral therapies.

MARRIAGE AS RISK, MARRIAGE AS REFUGE

Throughout Nigeria, Christians and Muslims alike stress the importance of marriage in fulfilling their religious obligations. At the same time, they emphasize its practical role in providing vital structures of economic and social support. Formal, arranged marriages are less common in urban northern Nigeria than they have been in the past. Nevertheless, it is not unusual for parents and other kin to introduce their daughters to potential spouses and to closely monitor their exchanges with suitors. Families almost always have the final say in their children's marital decisions. Nigerians widely believe marriage enables entire families to achieve upward social mobility.

In northern Nigerian marriages, men are expected to feel a sense of responsibility toward their wives and families, while women are supposed to display obedience toward their husbands. These unequal power arrangements are taken for granted as gender norms and are reinforced through social, religious, and even legal discourses. And yet, while these normative cultural expectations dictate that husbands must be able to economically support their families, many men cannot fulfill these demands.

Consequently, women make key contributions to household economies despite the fact that their labor is often hidden from view. By doing so, they garner authority in their relationships, while also protecting their husbands' reputations. With limited or inconsistent opportunities for sustainable incomes, however, women must often leverage their power to secure resources from others. For example, they may ask for loans from siblings, relatives, and other patrons. Or, they may offer loans and gifts to family members with the hope of receiving help at some point in the future.

The symbolic and material importance of marriage in northern Nigeria misleadingly suggests that women's partnerships with their husbands are durable and unchanging over time. In fact, these ties are highly fluid: a woman often circulates out of, and back into, a single marriage. She may also transition through a series of relationships over her life course.[9] Demographers report that Hausa-speaking Muslims have one of the highest divorce rates in the world.[10] Furthermore, women commonly marry much older men and become widows at young ages.[11]

The ease with which husbands can abandon and divorce their wives disinclines women from calling attention to their maltreatment. These acts include physical and emotional abuse, infidelity, and neglect. Without family members to back up their claims and provide them with financial support, women have a difficult time accessing the protections of the court system. When these marriages dissolve, their husbands and in-laws may deny them custody of their children, access to their possessions, and other rights guaranteed by religious and federal laws.

The study of kinship by Africanist anthropologists has a venerable history. Marriage plays a fundamental part of what scholars have called the "development cycle in domestic groups."[12] Families, they suggest, should be viewed as a process unfolding over time. They expand through practices such as marriage and reproduction to produce new generations. Then, they go through "fission" as members of a household separate to form their own families. And finally, the domestic group is replaced as parents die and children restore the original formation.

Kinship, however, entails more than just the rules that govern the reproduction of domestic groups. These social ties, scholars argue, also reveal relations of production.[13] Family members negotiate power and status through the allocation of rights and responsibilities according to age, gender, and other social divisions. Men acquire prestige and power by controlling the means of reproduction within their families. These include not only the exchange of subsistence goods but also the circulation of women through marriage.

Kinship plays a formidable role in laying out the ideological basis for social inequalities. In Nigeria, kinship norms are often underpinned by religious doctrines. They provide the justification for why the elderly should deserve the respect of the young and why men have control over women, among other cultural explanations for uneven relations of power. Anthropologists have proposed what they call wealth-in-people theory to further articulate the association between people's relationships and the reproduction of these unequal social structures.[14] In Africa, they describe, a person's status and influence depend directly on his or her ability to mobilize a following. While senior men acquire wealth and maintain their dominance through the control of women and junior men, young people may also receive symbolic and material benefits through strategic relationships with well-positioned patrons.

In northern Nigeria, many men are perpetually disenfranchised by the paucity of employment opportunities, low wages, and unrelenting obligations to kin. They cannot earn or save enough money to provide for the wives and families they desire. Married men, facing these same constraints, may seek out girlfriends or the possibility of new wives, through polygamous marriages, to save face and uphold their sexual reputations. Historically, scholars have documented how Nigerian wives would look the other way at signs of infidelity, so long as men are able to fulfill their family obligations.[15] In addition, Islam permits men to marry up to four wives. Many northerners believe women cannot prevent their husbands from marrying again if they are able to economically support their wives.

Anthropologists have noted how fundamentalist religious discourses condemning infidelity have intensified around the world, particularly through the spread of Evangelical and Pentecostal Christianity. Islamic religious leaders in northern Nigeria also proscribe extramarital affairs in public speeches, prayers, and texts, as well as television and radio broadcasts. As a result, men go to great lengths in order to hide their relationships. They are more likely to travel further away from their towns and solicit sex from strangers who will not expose their affairs to their communities, churches, or families.[16]

Women, too, are reluctant to confront their husbands, even if they know they are unfaithful. In a society that increasingly prizes marriages based on love as well as exchange, accusations of infidelity would lay bare the institution's contradictions and suggest women's marital relationships are indeed blighted. These allegations, whether expressed publicly or to their husbands alone, may lead to their divorce or abandonment.

Religious campaigns against infidelity in Nigeria often reference HIV as an imminent risk. Even so, most wives are unable to ask their husbands to use condoms. Such requests would imply that they know about the affairs and distrust their husbands. Married women, consequently, often deny they are at risk of HIV and remain silent about their husbands' extramarital relationships. These secrets, anthropologists have argued, exacerbate their likelihood of contracting the virus.[17]

While most Nigerians would attribute the spread of the HIV epidemic to unprotected sex among non-married youth, epidemiologists have shown that married women face an equal or greater risk of contracting HIV than their sexually active unmarried counterparts encounter. As I have found, treatment centers across the country are often filled with divorced and widowed women who have contracted HIV from their husbands. Indeed, in Nigeria, epidemiologists have added that *formerly* married (divorced, separated, or widowed) women have rates of HIV that double those who are currently married or cohabiting with a sexual partner.[18] While the epidemiological and social dynamics underpinning the relationship between HIV risk and marriage are increasingly well-understood, very little is known about how men and women reconstitute relationships after testing positive.

To understand why HIV-positive women seek refuge in (re)marriage when it was marriage that placed many of them at risk of the disease in the first place, this book adopts a processualist approach.[19] That is, rather than examining marriage as a discrete event established by clear legal, ritual, and economic transactions, I examine marriage as a process. I show how relationships are made and unmade through an array of practices and exchanges. For example, it is not unusual for women to have multiple suitors courting them simultaneously. They wait patiently to see which of these men will follow through on their romantic gestures with concrete plans and investments. Even prior to their formal wedding ceremonies, some women may call these men their "husbands," and the relationships may indeed resemble marriages in many ways.

Likewise, marriages may be undone through specific practices. For instance, Muslim Nigerian men use the flexibility of Islamic divorce proceedings to keep their options open. When divorcing a wife, they can choose to utter, "I divorce you" only one time, instead of saying it three times, allowing for the possibility of reconciliation at a later point in time. These women may be divorcees but only for a short period. There is not always a clear divide between married and nonmarried status among women. As HIV-positive women oscillate between these roles, much is at stake: on one hand, they may need to ask their families for help during these uncertain periods yet, on the other hand, they may have much to lose if their families learn their status.

ONE SECRET AMONG MANY

There are many ways to think about secrets and the roles they play in individuals' lives. Most commonly, secrets refer to private things, ideas, or experiences that escape recognition or knowledge by others. Implicit and explicit cultural guidelines direct our decisions to express certain things while withholding others. Often, people deliberately mask their thoughts because of the fearful or shameful consequences that potentially accompany their revelations. The act of hiding something may be done covertly through the use of disguise or concealment. In other cases, secrets may be out in the open: widely known but never spoken aloud – a public secret.[20] Psychologists commonly argue that secrets have a corrosive effect on a person's self-concept and social relationships. Therefore, identifying and disclosing these hidden sources of distress must be fundamental to the healing process.[21]

Anthropologists have countered that secrets may actually protect against social oppression and neutralize dangers. There is nothing inherent in a secret that suggests it is antisocial or unhealthy. On the contrary, secrets are fundamentally social; they both shape and are the products of social relations. Sharing secrets indexes preexisting qualities of social relationships, such as love, trust, and suspicion, while also accentuating hierarchical differences, such as who has the right to knowledge about others.[22]

Reflecting a broader movement in the field of anthropology at the end of the twentieth century, scholars have shifted their attention from social structures and formal linguistics to the role of secrecy in social interactions, exchange practices, and power dynamics. Too often, anthropologists have pointed out, the content of secrets is analyzed at the expense of the form through which secrets are (or are not) expressed. Anything can be declared a secret, regardless of how trivial or even fictitious. Members of a society may share this knowledge, but only some are permitted to speak about it. "The *contents* of the secrets are not as significant as the *doing* of secrecy," Beryl Bellman (1984) observes in her analysis of the Poro secret society in Liberia.[23] Likewise, Charles Piot (1993) concludes, "Secrecy seems not so much to hide something real, or exclude access to fixed things (wealth, status) as to set in motion a process – of interpretation, ambiguity, and the quest for hierarchy – and to keep it going."[24]

In contexts characterized by social upheaval, conflict, and profound economic and existential uncertainty, secrets proliferate. They exist in tandem with gossip, suspicion, and witchcraft accusations. Extended periods of ambiguity produced through secrecy enable individuals to protect themselves from false accusations – an ever-present fear, particularly in locales where structural inequalities routinely strip or undermine individuals' authority.[25] These scholars offer two important observations for this book: First, secrecy elevates the power attributed to concealed knowledge. And second, secrets provide a window into the relations of power that underscore how, when, and where knowledge is revealed.

This dynamic understanding of secrecy challenges the idea that secrets contain fixed, deeper meanings or truths imbued with emancipatory potential if revealed.[26] Secrets may not be hidden at all but rather partially known or revealed and constantly in negotiation among social actors. Indeed, if they are relegated exclusively to the domain of the unseen, then it would be nearly impossible for anthropologists to study them. "Secrecy," writes Michael Herzfeld (2009), "must itself be performed in a public fashion in order to be understood to exist" (135).[27]

One prominent assumption in Nigerian HIV counseling protocols is the idea that an HIV-positive diagnosis has a transformative effect on an individual's sense of self.[28] Physicians and counselors have told me that, upon learning their diagnosis, patients resolutely believe their deaths are imminent. Some blame themselves for contracting the virus. These counselors considered it their role to fix these erroneous assumptions. They suggested that while the public's attitudes and actions toward HIV-positive persons are harmful, the larger problem is that their clients stigmatize themselves by not talking about their status with others.

Drawing on his observations of HIV training workshops in Burkina Faso, medical anthropologist and physician Vinh-Kim Nguyen describes how "the process of being diagnosed with HIV was often recounted as a form of spiritual conversion, the first step on a road that led to greater enlightenment and the adoption of a more responsible, moral life."[29] He forcefully argues that HIV-positive persons' testimonials are much like commodities. Global development agencies employ them in their endeavors to secure funding for their respective programs. Few audiences questioned the "truth" behind these patients' salvation narratives. Rather, donors and patients alike were much more concerned with the social and economic resources for which these testimonials can be exchanged.

In the 1980s and 1990s, North American HIV-positive persons in gay communities effectively used AIDS testimonials in highly successful prevention campaigns. They were especially prominent in these activists' efforts to lobby the pharmaceutical industry for access to clinical trials and antiretroviral therapies.[30] As leaders of this social movement shared their strategies with global health agencies, they argued that highlighting the "face of AIDS" in Africa was a top priority. For one, these narratives offered proof that "AIDS is real" in contexts besieged by denialism and stigma. Second, they provided HIV-infected persons powerful tools to protest the inaction of developing country governments, which were either ill-equipped or unwilling to intervene in the epidemic. Nguyen refers to these efforts as "therapeutic citizenship" – that is, "a form of stateless citizenship whereby claims are made on a global order on the basis of one's biomedical condition."[31]

In ushering in programs that promoted "patient empowerment" through public speech, international and local organizations disrupted an existing set of predominantly kinship-bounded social relations that contributed to the survival of HIV-positive persons. They set into motion a new moral economy in which patient-activists exchanged testimonies with global donors for access to clinical trials. Those patients best able to tell a "good story" and develop rapport with these transnational professionals were most likely to access life-saving therapies.

My aim is not to diminish the significance of the political debates and successes of global HIV-positive activists, nor do I question the fact that there exist powerful incentives for being well-connected HIV-positive persons; indeed, my research has benefited immeasurably from these "professional" patients. In contrast to documenting a moral economy galvanized by the exchange of public testimonies, I focus instead on the currency of secrets. From her research among HIV-positive persons in Botswana, Jean Comaroff (2007) writes, "Maintaining the ambiguity of one's status, or the presence or absence of the disease, can be an act of self-preservation, defiance, or resignation in the face of an apparently implacable fate."[32] Women may conceal their status to actively deceive others and evade the virus's stigma; however, they may also conceal this knowledge because of the harm it would do to others.[33] Secrets index more than survival strategies. They also display respect, piety, and social distinction.

EVERYDAY ETHICS

Facing an overwhelming multitude of physical, social, and structural forms of violence, many HIV-positive women feel forced to the edge of the dignified values they strive to enact in their everyday lives. A positive diagnosis requires women to engage with both new and longstanding questions over how to live a meaningful life. These concerns, I suggest, are ethical matters.

In popular understandings of ethics, people often think about professional codes of conduct. For example, ethical review boards evaluate social scientists' research plans to ensure they protect their studies' participants. Ethics are commonly defined as the norms and obligations that constitute morality. According to this framing, ethics is a matter of following the rules. They provoke questions about the values that societies possess and whether humans are right to judge them for universal application or correctness. Ethics, when presented as such, are often problematically reduced to debates over cultural relativism. To avoid this pitfall, scholars frequently attempt to locate ethics in specific cases where clear violations of these principles become open to public debate. In these instances, the "right" thing to do is unknown. Questions of ethics materialize in human rights and legal debates, and through religious efforts to translate or transcend social breaches.[34]

The problem with this framework is that far too much analytical stress is given to ideals and the ability of humans to reason through these questions. It neglects motivation, desire, emotion, self-fashioning, comportment, and the ordinary sensibilities that people apply as they consider their conduct and the lives of others.[35] As humans aspire to behave ethically, they single out particular dimensions of their sense of self upon which to act. Further, they are subject to principles that legitimate or help them rationalize what they are doing. Because humans are always embedded in the lives of others, these aims and obligations also apply to exchanges within their social networks.

My focus in this book is on the ordinary, everyday ethics that constitute "living positively" (*rayuwar zaman lafiya*) with HIV – as Veena Das (2012) puts it, "the labor of bringing about an eventual everyday from within the actual everyday."[36] What actions do people take in the present to produce the futures they want? Specifically, I argue that care work is at the core of HIV-positive women's engagements in the realm of the ethical. I emphasize the labor that women devoted to the repair of their bodies and the bodies of others, the cultivation of intimate experiences, the generation of new and reliable modes of subsistence and exchange relations, and the mending, maintenance, and enhancement of their own and their families' reputations. In this text, I locate ethics in women's communication, bodies, and exchange practices.

If we define ethics as tacitly shared values and practices, it raises the question of how to identify these social facts. In other words, how do we hear what often goes unsaid? How do anthropologists observe "ordinary sensibilities" when women themselves do not necessarily identify or recognize them as such? First, as this book will show, ethics are embedded in our narratives and everyday conversations. Interviews, for example, are not unidirectional modes of communication. Just as in my exchange with Mary in the opening of this chapter, we ask each other questions, interrupt, translate, confirm, and express doubt, confusion, or outright disbelief. My interlocutors also used narratives to express and rework notions of morality. They attempted to create cogent explanations that I would understand, as well.[37]

These speech acts reveal more than just articulations of our thoughts and interior lives. They are also uttered in reference to publicly circulating discourses about morality, virtue, justice, and inequality. As described by Vinh-Kim Nguyen, in churches across West Africa, members of support groups testify that antiretroviral therapies allow them to be "born again" – comparing their bodily regeneration with a spiritual revival. These salvation metaphors enabled HIV-positive men and women to make sense of their experience and to persuade listeners that they are indeed living virtuous lives.

Anthropological investigations of communication stress that acts of speaking do more than convey meaning. They also serve performative functions. Speech is both a product of particular cultural contexts, as well as a means for transforming social structures. J. L. Austin (1965) offers the following classic example: if a pastor states, "I now pronounce you man and wife," to a couple in a church, he produces a new social reality. They are now married. When people speak, ethics is implicated in a myriad of ways: from the grammatical categories they employ to the patterns of interaction within conversations – such as the sequences of action that unfold, the configuration of participants, and the ways utterances are inflected by laughter, tears, emotions, and other unspoken and embodied gestures.[38]

Because HIV-positive women deeply fear the consequences of revealing their status to their partners and close relations, we can learn much about the intersection of speech and ethics by critically listening to how they evade disclosure. HIV-positive women use language to accomplish different things, such as to remove shame, to lend credibility to their experience, to express their anger and sense of violation, to seduce, and to communicate with God. In addition, by attending to the nuances of speech acts, anthropologists can consider how researchers participate in creating and reproducing these ethical engagements through interviews and everyday conversations.

Second, we can identify ethical practices not only through what people say and how they say it but also by what they do and when they do it. In other words, to live well, women not only talk about future hopes and dreams with others, but also labor upon their own bodies to produce this virtuous sense of self. Traditionally, anthropologists have theorized the body as a site where deeper cultural values are inscribed.[39] Among the HIV-positive women in the waiting rooms I described above, it was clear to me that their clothes did more than just cover their bodies. They symbolically revealed – or obscured – age, marital status, wealth, and religion, to name just a few.

Bodily adornments cement people's identities and make visible their social relations. For example, by wearing the conservative longer veils adopted by older, married women, young HIV-positive Muslims might project an image that meets local Islamic perceptions of modesty and virtue. They may simultaneously enhance their desirability among potential husbands.[40] Nevertheless, it is also important to consider what bodily practices like these *do* over simply what they mean. How, specifically, do these practices reproduce gender power dynamics?[41]

My focus in this text is thus on the ways women enact ethics through exchanges with their partners, families, neighbors, and health care professionals. Across the global health literature, public health scholars and practitioners document how young women's desires for fashion, jewelry, and other trendy items may lead them to pursue multiple sexual partnerships with older, wealthy men.[42] Intergenerational relationships, they argue, heighten their risk of contracting HIV. One prevention message in sub-Saharan Africa cautions women, "You might want the phone,

⌐ fancy clothes . . . But do you need HIV?" Nigerian political
⌐ous leaders also widely criticize the economic transactions be-
⌐n young women and their "sugar daddies," raising these same moral
objections.

There are numerous troubling assumptions in these behavioral change
campaigns and popular critiques of transactional sex and conspicuous
consumption. Most prominent among them is the idea that intimacy
is inimical to exchange; that is, the exchange of sex for money or gifts
debases love, sentiment, and religious virtue; it defiles the body; and it
reveals a lack of self-respect. Likewise, women's desires – beauty, social
experiences, and technology, for example – are distinct from and subordinate to their "real" needs. People's exchanges may, in fact, cement
gendered identities and social bonds. They animate a moral economy in
which objects and relationships become inextricably intertwined.

Exchange practices, just like women's bodily practices, are informed by
how women think about and attempt to shape their social networks and
their futures. Because women cannot predict the future or know what
these investments will ultimately produce, a narrow focus on the immediate utility that consumption provides obscures its other purposes. In
northern Nigeria, acts of giving and receiving also bestow virtue. Even
so, while gift-giving is often imbued with notions of equality and even
security, it is also fraught with dangers. These transactions can reveal deep-
seated social inequities, particularly in contexts of scarcity.

SECRECY AND ETHNOGRAPHY: RESEARCH METHODS

In July 2003, at the end of my first year of fieldwork, I stood with a group
of ten or so women and men at the front of a small Baptist church in Jos.
We sang a number of songs a counselor wrote for the support group. The
slight, yet startlingly charismatic physician and founder of the hospital
stepped forward with the microphone and introduced me to the congre-
gants: "And now our friend from America has a message for you." While
my face burned red from a combination of fear and embarrassment over
public speaking, I explained how increasing access to antiretroviral therapies was changing what it meant to live with HIV. Because of generous

funding from churches and other predominantly US-based charities, this hospital in Jos offered free HIV testing, counseling, and medications to prevent mother-to-child transmission. Donors also sent discarded drugs from American HIV-positive patients to the clinic. They were able to support a small number of men and women on the expensive triple cocktail of therapies. Within a year from my first visit, this hospital would be the first in Nigeria to access the free antiretroviral therapies offered by PEPFAR.

I had arrived at this clinic in the midst of a significant change in the course of the epidemic. At these church programs, we emphasized that HIV was no longer a death sentence. The passion and enthusiasm of the founder, staff, and many of the patients for HIV prevention and treatment were palpable. More people came each week for testing, and the nascent support group grew with each meeting.

After I spoke in these programs, a number of support group members would explain the mechanisms through which the virus is transmitted and ways to protect sexual partners. Others told stories about how they came to learn they had HIV and their experiences with the hospital. We concluded our "good will" messages with a plea for individuals to come forward for testing and for families and churches to show love and support for their HIV-positive members. Prayers and solicitations for donations followed these testimonies. Over the course of four months or so, I went to more than a dozen of these programs. Sometimes, we attended a church service in the morning and another in the evening. The support group shared the donations among its members. Those who gave personal testimonies received extra money.

At that time, I still, perhaps naively, believed the American assumption: "You are only as sick as your secrets." I thought that these public presentations and testimonies would have a transformative impact on both people's health and the broader epidemic. Indeed, it might even inspire political change. If Nigerians knew that HIV-positive persons were just like everyone else, then the fear and stigma would lessen. The government would be persuaded to invest greater money and resources into HIV treatment, hospitals, testing and counseling facilities, and social welfare programs to assist patients. Increasingly, HIV-positive support group members could obtain economic benefits through support groups, such as occupational training in sewing, knitting, farming, or other trades; paid positions in the hospital or "volunteer" experiences that could allow them to secure jobs in other clinics; help with other health care needs, such as prenatal care and baby formula; travel opportunities; and friendships with the hospital's wealthy patrons.

And yet, as a participant in these programs, I learned that some of the group members were ambivalent or even reluctant to take part in public events. They said that they needed the money, but disliked having to spend so much time and energy going to all of these events. Some were noticeably uncomfortable sharing their experiences with strangers. It also became clear that the stories they would tell me in interviews were not the same as those they delivered in churches. At the same time, Mary and other HIV-positive women's desires to marry and have children intrigued me. I suspected that these concerns referenced a much more important anthropological question: how has the HIV epidemic transformed kinship ties, and in what ways have these realignments shaped HIV-positive women's access to social and economic resources?

To answer this question, I needed to understand more about how kinship networks and exchange relationships intersect in Nigeria. After spending ten months in Jos that year, I moved to the city of Kano in the far north of the country to continue my project. At first sight, Kano was strikingly different from Jos. Walking down the street, the prominence of Islam was evident in the ubiquitous mosques across the city and the muezzins' stirring, melodic calls to prayer five times a day. Businesses display photographs and paintings of men and women in traditional Hausa clothes, selling everything from mobile phones to traditional medicines.

Kano is not only the capital of Kano State, with its booming population of over 10 million, but it is also considered the cultural, religious, and economic center of Hausa-speaking Nigeria. The city's history dates back over a thousand years. Its residents include Muslims and a minority of Christians from all parts of the country. Kano State was also distinct because of its total fertility rate: women in Kano have on average more than eight children, which nearly double the rates of other regions in the country.

My host during my first three-month long trip to Kano in 2004 was a journalist. She introduced me to the president of a nongovernmental organization (NGO) that sponsored HIV education programs, counseling and testing, and a support group for persons living with HIV. I met this woman in her office in the back of one of northern Nigeria's oldest public health schools where she taught. I described my project and my observations from Jos about women's desire to marry and have children. Although she seemed surprised and a little suspicious of my research goals, she took out her phone and requested that Hauwa, a member of the support group, come to her office to meet me. Hauwa assembled a group of around ten women with whom I could work. The NGO offered us their headquarters to hold my meetings. I conducted interviews in a large, carpeted room, which was empty apart from several upholstered wooden chairs and a few scattered posters and calendars hung on the walls.

One day later that summer, I entered the office and found a large group of women gathered in its conference room. The NGO was holding a meeting that afternoon. They pointed me to a storage closet where I could talk to women in private that day. A number of the other HIV-positive women with whom I worked came to participate in the program. In the middle of my interview, I was interrupted by one of them. The meeting had recently adjourned, and she was annoyed. This woman said that the organization wanted to make a calendar with members' pictures to promote HIV prevention. I could tell that she felt good about standing up to the organization's leaders and refusing to be photographed. However, this woman was clearly nervous about the consequences of declining their request. She then asked if we could change the venue of my interviews to a different office.

Just a few blocks away stood a building that housed another support group's office. The women invited me to attend their monthly meeting, which was held that weekend. I was struck by the program's formality. There were no intimate discussions about their health or any of the other issues women had raised in their conversations with me over the past month. In fact, no one even disclosed their HIV status, much less brought up relationship dilemmas. Although women dominated the group's membership, most remained silent while the men discussed their fundraising efforts and concerns about replacing one of their officers.

Confused, I returned to my weekly meeting with these women and asked them, "Why would you join groups that offer you so little help and whose publicity potentially threatens to expose your status?" I learned that many of these women welcomed their assistance, however meager, but they had little interest in participating in education programs or outreach. Women felt they had too much to lose if their communities learned they were HIV positive. I probed them further, and it soon became evident that women did not join the group for psychosocial support; they joined to meet potential husbands.

In fact, the group's leaders played an active role in "match making." They even provided a small cash gift when their couples married. Once married, many women left the support group. Because HIV was seen by the public to be largely a disease that affected unmarried women and widows, few would guess that a new bride could also be HIV positive. Northern Nigerian women "go public" by joining support groups so that they might marry, reconstitute their families, and, in turn, secure their privacy.

Between 2004 and 2014, I made eight trips to northern Nigeria, lasting in duration from a few weeks to ten months. I spent the majority of my time in Kano, with occasional trips to Jos, Abuja, and other cities across the north. In Kano, I lived in the suburb of Hotoro with a shorter period of time inside the "old city" neighborhood of Chedi. In addition, I resided with families in Gyadi-Gyadi, Bompai, and Shagari Quarters – all densely populated areas of this urban state capital.

Much of my day-to-day life in Kano centered on the activities of these different families. I would accompany them to their workplaces, markets, schools, relatives' and friends' homes, parties, weddings, condolences visits, and other formal occasions. I watched, for example, how men and women interacted with each other, what they talked about, and how people participating in the weddings described the process of courtship and marriage. Through my hosts inside the old city, I met a "matchmaker" in their neighborhood who introduced me, in turn, to a number of widows and divorcees in Chedi and the surrounding areas, most of whom were her clients and friends. With these individuals, I conducted approximately fifty semistructured interviews on an array of issues related to their family life and marriage dissolutions.

I also collected in-depth interviews from more than eighty HIV-positive women, focusing primarily on the people I met from my first two visits and introductions to their friends. Two-thirds of these women were married at least once. Although most of them resided in Kano State at the time of our interviews, many grew up in states across Nigeria. The majority of women spoke Hausa as their native language, and they were raised in Muslim families. However, at least twenty-five of those I interviewed were Christian or were raised in Christian families. Northern Nigerians commonly learn English as their second or third language. Some of the women in my study could speak English conversationally while others spoke it fluently. The latter was especially the case if they attended secondary schools or universities where English was the language of instruction. Others spoke English because they had resided outside of the north, where English or Pidgin English was the lingua franca. As I carried out these interviews in both English and Hausa, I often worked closely with two research assistants, who spoke Hausa, Yoruba, and English and could translate when needed. We communicated in the language with which women felt most comfortable.

As I learned in my first trips to Nigeria, conversations about HIV are universally hard. They span references to physiological, emotional, and social suffering; gendered violence; family abandonment; child death; and poverty, to name just a few. I thus conducted interviews with what scholars have called an ethnographic imaginary – that is, with a goal of understanding the cultural context of individuals' lives. In short, rather than limiting interviews to the immediate research questions, this approach probes for a wide range of details about people's lives and the social milieu they inhabit.

Interviews might begin with general questions such as the following: What characterizes a beautiful woman? Or, tell me about why it is so difficult for women to save money? Alternatively, I might start with more personal open-ended questions, such as, "Tell me about yourself." I would turn to biographical information, such as their descriptions of childhood, families, and schooling, followed by adolescence, relationships, and marriage.

If the conversations were going well, I would ask more detailed questions about interpersonal conflicts, sicknesses, and the dissolutions of marriages. I reviewed with them their relationship ideals and how women go about marrying again. I often concentrated on the social significance of childbirth and children, as well as the importance of family relations in influencing men and women's relationship trajectories.

I almost never initiated interviews with questions about HIV. I waited instead for my informants to bring it up in our conversations. These

discussions spanned issues related to HIV and the life course: their experiences in knowing or caring for HIV-positive persons, prevention efforts,
potential exposure(s) to the virus, social stigma, complications with sexual
functions and fertility, medications, and HIV-related morbidity and mortality. In conjunction with these interviews, I conducted a survey and
completed event history calendars with 100 HIV-positive women, charting
the households in which they have lived since their first marriage. These
women came from three different support groups and four different hospitals across the city.

Over this same period, I also observed the day-to-day operations
of an HIV treatment center, where initially, approximately 250 men and
women collected antiretroviral therapies. This figure has now grown
to more than a thousand adults and children. I attended staff meetings,
pretest and posttest counseling sessions, and training workshops. I also
informally spent time with doctors, nurses, laboratory technicians, phar-
macists, and other people involved in the clinical management of HIV.
Within the counseling sessions, I listened to the advice patients were given
regarding their changes in health, treatment, adherence, sexuality, fertility, and preventive behaviors, as well as the concerns that patients raised.

I was particularly interested in how patients reflected upon HIV-related
illnesses and fatalities as well as the influence of antiretrovirals and their
side effects on their daily life activities. I observed how they were recruited
into this treatment program and the hospital staff's efforts to encourage
them to return for follow-up care and medications. One of the HIV-
positive women I interviewed in 2004 – and my closest friend and key
informant – was a counselor who I shadowed not only at the hospital but
also through much of her daily life over numerous visits. More than any
other individual, her case and understandings about HIV-positive women's
experiences have informed many of the arguments I make in this book.

The nature of my exchanges with HIV-positive women also changed
during the latter period of my research. Although I continued to immerse
myself in the lives of the same women with whom I worked earlier in my
study, I concentrated less on formal, tape-recorded interviews with these
individuals. Instead, our interactions were much more informal. Because
I maintained relationships with these women for many years, some eventually became comfortable with me accompanying them to their homes.
I spent time with them as they cooked and cared for their children. We

would shop and visit their relatives. Mostly, we gossiped about boyfriends and marriages, news about people we knew in common, and our own critical thoughts on women's social position, the abuses of family members, our misgivings about treatment programs and support groups, and Nigerian politics more generally.

My interest in support group politics and dynamics waned during these years. In part, this was because their meetings became so large that they were mainly centered on lectures. More significantly, many of the women I first met in these groups had themselves lost interest in attending meetings. Some maintained their relationships with the group leaders and NGOs and could call upon them if they had urgent needs. Others would occasionally agree to participate in programs that might give them money or other resources. And, of course, they would try to stay in touch with the friends they made there. But mostly, these women had other work and social obligations they had to meet. Consequently, I followed them as they moved beyond their support groups.

LEADING STORIED LIVES

Anthropologists are well aware of the fact that our informants' personal accounts do not exist in a vacuum. We collaborate with our interlocutors as we share stories with one another and answer each other's questions. While my interviews were most often conducted in private settings, the presence of other actors inside and outside the rooms in which we spoke also contoured the narratives they offered me. These people included my research assistants, the counselors who introduced us, the directors and staff of the clinics and NGOs, and, undoubtedly, the people that women themselves imagine would listen to or read their stories. For instance, although my initial interview questions rarely touched on HIV, women knew from the very beginning – from the fact that our conversations took place in an HIV clinic or support group and from my years of doing this work with their friends and fellow patients, as two of many cues – that I wanted to learn more about their diagnosis.

My sensitivity toward the social position I occupied in these exchanges and relationships reflects one of the hallmarks of ethnographic research and writing. For some women, I was a curious foreigner with whom they spoke for a short period while waiting to collect medications from their physician. To many, I suspect that I was no different from the legions of foreign researchers, public health practitioners, and clinicians who also visit the clinics and support groups they attended. For others, I was a regular visitor who returned annually to greet them and talk about the events of the preceding year. They also knew intimate details about my personal life. Just as I paid close attention to their physical and social changes, so too did they observe how I matured as a scholar and a person over the course of a decade.

Throughout the text, my presentations of women's stories – in their own words, through translation, or summarized by me – have been attentive to the questions and context that provoked these responses. And, in my interpretations of their meanings and the larger social patterns to which they refer, I have tried to be careful about the limits of what I can say about any particular woman's case. No one can know an individual's life entirely. Certainly, this cannot be ascertained in a series of interviews or even in years of friendship. In some narratives, I have expressed explicitly my confusion or doubt. In others, I have noted what such stories *could* mean or what they reveal more broadly about the person or to other similarly situated women.

To contextualize the descriptions I collected from HIV-positive women, I relied on triangulation, the primary tool that anthropologists use to make larger social and cultural interpretations. This means that we evaluate all of the different kinds of data we have gathered to make sense of what we have written in our notes, heard in our interviews, and observed in the field. For each woman whose story you read here, I have worked with dozens more, who offered very similar and very different accounts. This allowed me to compare their cases, teasing out what appear to be common trends and singular phenomena. Through surveys, I learned about women's backgrounds, attitudes, decisions, and values in the aggregate. Through participant observation, I watched women's dilemmas and decisions unfold in real time – in clinics, workplaces, households, and other settings where they go about the business of living their lives. Moreover, these interviews, surveys, and observations took place among HIV-positive and HIV-negative women, alike, as well as their families and friends.

Nevertheless, there are limits to the materials I use in this book. The most prominent of my omissions is the lack HIV-positive men's narratives.

You will learn only one side of these deeply gendered concerns. I did not conduct these interviews for a number of reasons. First, I began my research within HIV support groups where women greatly outnumbered men. Many of them were the current or former partners of the women I interviewed. These women undoubtedly would have been suspicious about what men told me and, perhaps more problematically, what I shared with them, whether true or not. Because my conversations were usually about women's husbands and boyfriends, it would have been awkward for me to ask them to meet and interview their partners.

As I expanded my research from support groups into HIV treatment centers, there was a much larger population of men; however, I was doubtful that they would want speak to me, as a woman, especially given that my questions related to sexuality, money, and other deeply moral matters. Northern Nigerian women know all too well that men regularly deceive them over the very issues that I study. They warned me repeatedly that HIV-positive men lie, and I could not trust the stories they tell. I initially conceded this point at its face value.

And yet, it was also not lost on me that many of these women could not confront their partners directly about their duplicitous behavior. I suspect now that their efforts to discourage me were also an informal way of reclaiming that sense of power through a performance of secrecy. I, in turn, contributed to that effort by refraining from interviewing men and withholding what I knew about them. Thus, I not only heard about people's secrets but also participated in the performance of secrecy over the course of my research.

For the women in my study, this book embodies a public secret. It contains things that are widely known among HIV-positive and HIV-negative people, alike, but rarely spoken about. These women were fully aware that their narratives would be presented in the text and read by unknown others, and yet my promise of anonymity meant the content of these secrets would not be entirely exposed, nor would the fact that they are the authors of these accounts. Through our conversations, women invited me to learn more about the things they wanted me to know; still, they withheld descriptions of other aspects of their lives. This enabled them to retain authority over their carefully concealed knowledge. In exchange, I respected these boundaries and the limitations of their individual perspectives.

Some of the narratives you will read are frustratingly incomplete. Just as I described in my interview with Mary, many of these stories meander back and forth in time. They go off on tangents and cease at places that beg for further elaboration. Others, I found, were riddled with contradictions and claims that even I doubted – although I could never be sure. These halting, circuitous, and sometimes misleading narratives reveal more than simple miscommunications or poorly structured questions. Women's silences, lies, and exaggerations not only illuminate subversions of power but also raise important questions about how these individuals make sense of their lives, present themselves as ethical persons, and reframe fragmented recollections of suffering and survival into evidence of a more hopeful future.

1

First Loves

"When I was a very young woman, men would compliment me a lot!" Amira, a married woman from Kano in her twenties, described to me:

> When they said I was beautiful, I felt as if I was on top of the world. I felt so happy and proud among my friends. Then came my future husband, John. He kept on pursuing me . . . it was just a "boyfriend and girlfriend" routine. He would wait on the road outside my house to take me to school. . . . He was twenty-eight years old and I was a just a young girl. Let's say around thirteen. He knew that lots of young guys were after me – younger than him. Good-looking guys! He dedicated a lot of time to me so that I would not escape from him. He would take me home after school. His car would be parked right at the school gate. I remember how my principal – who liked me so much – put me on suspension because of this. I was young and intelligent. She did not think John would allow me to focus on school. She thought I was too young for so much attention.

I asked Amira, "How did John show you that he really loved you?" And she responded, "He showered me with a lot of gifts." I prompted her to tell me more. She paused and then continued:

> He gave me a wristwatch and then one of those handmade cards by artists. Very big! My picture was inside with loving words and hearts . . . I took it to school. When my friends saw it, everybody said it looked so amazing: "This man really loves you!" Then, later on, he bought shoes and clothing. He bought cultural wears [cloth] and he sent a tailor to me. The tailor

would come to my house, measure me, and sew different dresses. Shoes, bags, wristwatches, bangles . . . and money! From time to time, he gave me 2,000 naira [$14].

"Just 2,000?" I teased, knowing that this was a lot of money for a young woman to receive from her boyfriend. "Then, 2,000 naira was so much!" She answered:

> I became the "big girl" in school. Everybody was jealous. My friends and I were eating different kinds of sweets and drinks with his money. We ate snacks so that everyone could see we were rich. . . . In my family, I am not from a very big [rich] background, so I did not hide from them the gifts he showered on me. I would give the money to my mother: "Mommy, this is what this guy gave me and these are the gifts." At times, my mother would say, "Open them and share with your sisters."

In the context of Nigeria's HIV epidemic, much attention has been paid to the sexual activities of young people. Men and women between the ages of fifteen and twenty-four account for the majority of cases of HIV on the African continent. Furthermore, young women are more likely to be infected than men. Their disproportionate vulnerability to HIV, scholars have argued, results primarily from unequal gender power relations. They reflect the larger structural inequalities that obstruct people from pursuing safe, mutually faithful relationships. Women may lack the flexibility to make choices or demands on their sexual partners. Older men, in particular, may pressure them into having sex, and their need for money and gifts from boyfriends – their "sugar daddies" – can exacerbate these power imbalances. Such constraints are not only a product of economic inequalities. Religious and cultural norms, which assert that virtuous women must be deferential in their interactions with boyfriends, further affect their ability to protect themselves from HIV.

While these analyses outline crucial social forces shaping the epidemic around the world, epidemiologists' broad brushstrokes cannot capture the complex meanings and motivations surrounding intimacy and sex among youth.[1] Through a series of stories that women have told me about their first relationships, I aim to offer a window into young Nigerians' strategies for navigating desire and love. All of the women in this chapter ultimately tested HIV positive. Few know from whom or when, precisely, they became infected by the virus. My goal here, however, is not to trace the explicit factors that led each of these particular women to contract HIV. Rather, I will show the ways women's negotiations and assertions of agency are caught up in the structural forces that reproduce social inequalities.

As Amira's story above shows, one prominent theme in women's accounts of their adolescent love lives is the ways in which intimacy and exchange are intertwined. Money and gifts play a key role in men's displays of their affection and attraction. They may also express their sincerity and ability to marry. *Kudin zance*, literally meaning "discussion money" in Hausa, is almost always expected in routine visits from male suitors. They might offer a soft drink, cookies, or candy. It could also be a small amount of money or other token gift. Wealthier men may give larger items such as cloth, jewelry, or even cell phones. There are not always clear distinctions between the money men give women for sex and other kinds of material exchanges between sexual partners in intimate relationships.

None of the women I met over the course of my ten years in northern Nigeria would say they had sex with "clients" for money, distancing themselves from the partnerships of sex workers. They called their partners "boyfriends" and referred to themselves as their "girlfriends." Many knew women that they would identify as hustlers or prostitutes, however. Although rarely openly discussed, houses of *karuwai* (the Hausa term for prostitutes) were once common across the north. The reinstitution of *Shari'a* criminal law in northern states has intensified political and religious efforts to close these houses. Nevertheless, most northern Nigerians will point out that rich and poor men alike easily locate sex workers in areas where *Shari'a* restrictions are relaxed as well as nearby cities, such as Kaduna or Abuja.[2] Sexual affairs between young women and older married men are carefully hidden but common across the north, just as they are across the country and the continent. These relationships may involve exchanges of substantial amounts of money.

Teachers and parents often pressure young women to focus on their studies and not romance. And yet, for some of them, sexual partnerships with men may actually be part of their plans to advance academic and career goals. In Nigerian popular culture, stories abound of women's relationships with a "Mr. Lecturer." Sometimes, they feature professors who coerce young women into having sex with them for higher grades. In others, women are the seductresses. The cunning attitudes and ways in which men and women extract emotional, sexual, and material resources from each other are common themes across a variety of media from sensationalistic newspaper accounts to films and music. Audiences both laud and denounce them as fundamentally "Nigerian" aspects of people's love lives.[3]

Gifts are not static expressions of a man's love, however; they also produce affection and pleasure.[4] A gift of jewelry, for example, allows a man to admire a woman's beauty. As he slips a ring on his girlfriend's finger, he might touch her hands in a deeply sensual way. Another man might give his girlfriend money to go to the salon and style (*plait*) her hair. Or, like Amira's boyfriend, he may pay for a tailor to sew a dress that he thinks will complement her attractiveness. Women prize gifts of cell phones and call credit in part because they let couples speak in private, out of reach of prying ears.[5] Women cautioned me not to reduce their intimate experiences to sex alone. Sex is one act among an array of exchanges and experiences that they hope will potentially lead to marriage.

Although marriage remains a critical goal for Christians and Muslims alike, the duration of time before young women actually wed has grown in recent years. A number of factors have contributed to this change, including the high cost of weddings, increasing access to higher education, and young women and men's desires for marriages with greater independence from their respective families. Religious leaders and community elders decry upward trends in premarital sex within this period of protracted adolescence in northern Nigeria. Family members intensely scrutinize young women's courtships. Parents may withhold information about contraception and reproduction from their daughters because they believe this knowledge will only further motivate them to have sex. Indeed, most northerners speak about sex in idiomatic terms rather than with explicit terminology, such as the "meeting" between men and women. Young women deeply fear accusations of defiance, greed, or immoral behavior. Furthermore, if their parents learn they have been sexually active, they face much greater sanctions than young men would. Family elders still play formidable roles in determining whether marriages can proceed.

Young men and women not only navigate the need to hide their relationships from their elders; they also hide many things from one another. A man may be married without his girlfriend's knowledge. He may borrow a car from a friend or even wear someone else's clothes when he visits her. He may lie about his job, income, and family. Women say that men are skilled in hiding their true marriage intentions. And they, in turn, hide stories of past relationships, sexual and reproductive experiences, and health issues, among other kinds of information. Women may also lie about their families, education, and homes to cover up the poverty in which they were raised. Few are candid about their desires, as well – especially if they have no interest in marrying these particular boyfriends.

While these acts of deception may seem like serious moral violations undermining the pursuit of "true" love, women know their partners are never fully honest with them. In fact, a woman would be taken aback if a man told her all of his shortcomings up-front. "It would never happen!" one of my friends said with a loud laugh when I asked her this exact question. If a man had no money or was looking for work, for example, she might feel compelled to help him. And yet, I heard countless stories about women who loaned their boyfriends money, only for these men to abandon them as soon as they received it. If a woman knows from the beginning that her prospective boyfriend is incapable of supporting her, she may reject him before they grow too close. However, if she learns these details after their relationship has matured, she might respond sympathetically. This same friend responded that she would then think seriously about whether she could still marry the man despite his flaws.

Women are also reluctant to share too many details about their personal lives when they first meet suitors. They fear men will use this information for malicious purposes. While their apprehension hints at larger inequalities, stories of deception may also be extremely funny. This "dance" between concealment and exposure is a normal experience among young people negotiating love and loss in northern Nigeria. In what follows, I trace women's efforts to project an image of respectability while exercising discretion in their exchanges with men.[6]

CELINE

Gifts solidify social ties as part of specific spoken and unspoken exchanges between men and women. A man's relentless efforts to demonstrate his generosity to a woman he admires and her tacit acceptance of his gifts and attention reveal their mutual interest in one another.

Women demonstrate their respectability through displays of timidity or shame (*kunya*). Shyness, in other words, is not necessarily a sign of their disinterest. During the summer of 2010, I met with a young woman named Celine. She was twenty-six years old and a Christian, originally from Bauchi State. Her narrative about the first time a young man proclaimed his love to her highlights these silent dynamics.

Celine began:

> There was this time when I was young – just after starting secondary school. I was at boarding school. At the end of every month, families come and visit the students. So one guy entered the school. As I was walking to see my mother, he spotted me. He asked his younger sister, who was in my class, to get my attention. . . . When I approached him, he said he just saw me passing and that he was in love with me.

I asked Celine what she did about this. She said:

> I was ashamed! It was the first time a boy talked to me . . . I told him, I am coming back. Then I ran away! I went back to the hostel where I lived and thought about it some more . . . I reconsidered and said, 'Okay.' When the guy's sister came back, she brought me some money from her brother . . . I said that I did not want it and that she should return it to him.

"How much?" I asked. She thought for a moment, "That time it was 200 naira [$1.50]." I pressed her, "Was that a lot of money?"

> It was a lot of money for a student. Then, over the next visiting day, the boy came again. He sent for me and I went to see him. He talked to me, but I could not say anything in response. I was so shy.

"How did he show you that he loves you? What did he say? What did he do?" I wanted to know.

> He was a photographer. He snapped pictures of me and printed some of them. He gave me his own picture, too. When he came to see me, he would buy me something . . . like juice, sweets, and so on. When I saw those things, I would be happy. There were other gifts, like money, and beautiful accessories such as bags, head ties, and shoes.

"So then what happened to him?" I followed up.

> Once, he called me to his house. I went to see him and his father was at home. His father saw me, but he did not say anything. He took me into his

room and we sat, again, just 'gisting' [chatting]. Then, the guy said, for the first time, that he wanted to do something. I refused because I was a virgin. I left the house. I was afraid. . . . He continued to come to my house to see me, but I did not go to his house again. I just did not know what would happen there.

Like most women, Celine began her story of her first love by describing how her boyfriend found her. Surprised that men would just follow girls they admired without knowing anything about them, I asked another woman to explain. She said, if a man sees an attractive woman, he might ask around to see if anyone knows her. He will describe what she looks like, and her neighbors may give him her address. In other instances, one of his friends might give him the number and address of a girl he should meet and he will attempt to locate her. Women hesitate to acknowledge men's attention – initially running away or even denying their gifts, in Celine's case. Most people, in fact, would read these passive communication and body practices as a display of her good character or upbringing.

One-sided conversations, where men talk while women listen, are not uncommon. In fact, by declining to speak to this suitor, I think Celine implied that she *was* interested in him. "Whatever he says," one friend told me, "is cool by her." The man might begin by telling her, "I like you," and then ask her a few questions. If she is afraid to speak, she would say quickly, "No, you first." The man would give details about himself: the place where he currently lives and where he was born. He could describe his work, such as the name of the business or organization. If he works in a market, he might say what he sells and where he travels. He would also tell her about his family, such as how many siblings he has and whether he was the first or last born or somewhere in the middle.

After speaking for a while, he might ask her again to tell him about herself. If she still does not want to talk, he would continue to ask her questions and she could just nod or shake her head. He might then invite her to have lunch with him. A quiet, young woman like Celine would probably not agree to go initially. But, she would accept gifts, such as juice or biscuits, and thank the young man. She would then show off these items to her friends and they would gossip for hours about him. Gifts provide women the first sign that their boyfriends have feelings for them.

Many women I know claim that they were not aware of their boyfriends' sexual intentions while they were first being courted. Nonetheless, most acknowledged that young men were also motivated to find partners with whom they could have sex. Thus, while Celine claimed to be surprised by her boyfriend's sexual advance in his room, I still suspect that she knew or had a sense that physical intimacy was a possibility, if she expressed interest.

When I discussed this woman's story with others, they identified a number of signs that could have revealed the young man's sexual motives to Celine. Most importantly, they raised the following question: why would the father remain silent as his son passed him by with a woman? No respectable man would watch his son bring girls into his room without intervening or at least introducing himself. Perhaps the son paid for the household bills or rent, they speculated, which could mean that his father has no grounds to challenge his behavior. Or possibly, the father already fought with the son over this issue and they were not speaking to one another. In other words, it meant he brought other women into his room. These women surmised that Celine was likely as alarmed by the father's behavior as she was by the son's advance. That is why she must have run away, they said. Her boyfriend, nevertheless, continued to pursue her. Nigerian men, my one friend repeated, do not give up until they get what they want.

PATIENCE

Patience is one of my closest friends and key informants in Kano. One afternoon, a group of us had an animated conversation about the power lecturers have over their students. Specifically, we discussed their ability to intimidate young women into sexual relationships by threatening to fail them. Everyone was quick to condemn the behavior of these men. Patience interjected, "But these university students are also corrupt!"

Patience then told us about her experience as a young woman employed at a restaurant on a university campus in Kaduna State. Her aunt, who managed the restaurant, was a very smart woman. She warned Patience that she should be careful because men would come to the restaurant just to see her. Patience described how some men would buy a soft drink for themselves and then pay her 100 naira, which was over four times the actual price of a Coca-Cola at that time. They would tell Patience to keep the change and buy herself a drink.

Patience recounted a story about a 300-level (third-year) engineering student, who regularly came to visit her at the restaurant. This young Yoruba man would bring her money and other small gifts. He told Patience that he was in love with her. She would respond to him that she was thinking it over. One time, she took a motorcycle (taxi) home and he followed her. He waited for Patience outside her gate. When she entered the house, her cousins told her that a man was there to see her. Patience was surprised to see him. He said he wanted to know where she lived. She protested and asked him to go. Patience finally said that she was not interested.

Then, Patience was around 20 years old and saving money for school. While she did want to marry, it was not the right time. Patience said that while many of her admirers also brought other girlfriends to the restaurant to try and make her jealous, he never would. Even when he bought sodas for the women at his table, he assured Patience that these women were his classmates, not girlfriends. She found his generosity and honesty to be charming.

As she recounted this story about the young man, Patience seemed wistful. He was not the "corrupt" character to which she was referring when we began our discussion. Rather, he was one persistent man in a series of men who sought her attention when she was young. If she got married, she explained, she would not be able to return to school. The benefit of extra income from a boyfriend was not worth the risk, she thought. Patience eventually grew accustomed to the attention she received from young men around campus, although she hastily added that she was still afraid of them.

Among the patrons of the restaurant, she knew that there were differences between men with good and bad intentions. She learned how to speak evasively, occasionally collecting their gifts and money, but refusing to commit to going out with them. Like Celine's suitor, the man above located her house, and expressed his love for her. I told Patience that, from my perspective, his insistence was disingenuous. "He barely knew anything about you!" I said. She responded, "Well, I do not really know," but she thought his reluctance to bring girlfriends to the restaurant was an indication of his love. Eventually, he moved away and she did not see him again. He was far from the last of her admirers.

Patience told me about another man who also visited her in the restaurant. He was in the same academic year as the other admirer, but lived in a different hostel. At first, he wrote her a note telling her his name and that he was in love with her. When Patience met him at the restaurant, she asked him, "What do you mean by this?" He repeated what he wrote to her and then asked, "Well, what do you think?" And, like the man above, Patience said to give her time. She would think about it.

This guy, Patience described, was very rich and would buy her expensive things. She exclaimed, "Hey!" to emphasize both her surprise and approval as she listed these gifts to me. One time, he came up to the restaurant in his car and offered to give Patience a ride. He wanted her to see his room at the hostel. She quickly responded no. Patience explained to him she had to work late that evening. So, he wrote down his room number on a piece of paper and said she should come after she closed. Patience crumbled up the paper and threw it away. Another time, he brought his parents to the restaurant and introduced her. "This is the woman I want to marry," he said to them. Patience was surprised by his introduction but then dismissed it as another extravagant gesture to convince her to sleep with him.

Sure enough, when he returned the next day to the restaurant, he asked her, "Why didn't you come to see me last night?" Patience explained to him that her aunt came to pick her up and she could not visit him. She then told him again she was not interested. Finally, Patience asked the man to leave. Eventually, she said, she just had to quit her job at the restaurant because of this attention.

Both Patience's and Celine's ability to speak to men without overtly implying interest – saying "I will think about it" or even lying – reveals strategies for maneuvering around men's relentless propositions. By labeling men in universities as "corrupt," Patience suggested that these young students primarily want sexual, not marital, relationships. Furthermore, she emphasized that gifts alone do not signify a man's good intentions; this was not love. In fact, gifts are potentially deceptive. And yet, as Patience stepped back to reflect on her first admirer's character, she appreciated his effort to assure her that he was not pursuing multiple girlfriends. She closely watched his behavior at the restaurant and even seemed to reconsider her initial charge about the poor character of men in universities. Like many women in her position, she felt conflicted. She wanted to pursue her degree, but she could not entirely ignore the attention men paid to her. Still, Patience neither wanted to sleep with these men nor was she ready to marry.

ASAMA'U

Asama'u, a young Muslim woman from Kano State, was twenty-six years old when I first met her. In an interview about how she became infected with HIV, she paused on the description of her first boyfriend – the first man she loved:

> As soon as I began to have feelings for my boyfriend, I started hating school.... He sent his relatives to our house to ask for my hand in marriage. My parents told his people that it was not possible – that I would finish school first. At the time, he was twenty-five and I was thirteen. My parents told him they did not like him and he should stop coming to see me. After his second attempt and failure to get my parents' permission . . . we went to the *mallam* [an Islamic healer] who promised us help. What I fail to understand, even up until today, is: how come the love we felt for each other became so intense after our visit to him? Of course, we were taking love potions from the *mallam* and there were items he ordered to be buried. My boyfriend took care of that, since it is the man's responsibility. After that, things changed. In the past, I did not spend much time visiting with him. Now, I would stay at his house until after 11 p.m., talking to him. At the time, he was much more mature than me. He would say, "Let me adjust your head tie," or some other excuse to hold my hand. Or, he would buy me a ring and put it on my finger. We would meet whenever I went out to watch movies at a friend's house.

When Asama'u was a child, social attitudes towards education underwent a shift toward the importance of "girl child education" in northern Nigeria. Her parents' insistence on her remaining in school, at least in part, reflects the changes ushered in by Universal Primary Education policies in the 1970s. Even with this change, early marriage in the north is common, and Asama'u resented the fact that she was not permitted to wed this man when other friends were already married. Some young women will marry and resume their schooling, while their husbands assume the costs of their school fees. Although her parents may have refused to allow Asama'u to marry because of their education goals for her, their reasons could equally have had to do with the boyfriend's character.

In this case, Asama'u and her boyfriend attempted to charm her parents into allowing them to wed by seeking the advice of a *mallam* – an Islam scholar who applies his knowledge of the traditions of the Qur'an and the hadith to heal people suffering from a diverse range of spiritual, social, and physiological problems. The healing techniques may involve a "potion" made from a solution upon which the healer has prayed. They may also include consuming "washed" texts inscribed with verses of the Qur'an. Other techniques involve burying items or substances that are blessed.

These charms, Asama'u believed, let them spend time alone together until late into the night without her parents' knowledge. She thought the potions and rituals only targeted her parents' attitude toward him. So, it came as a surprise to Asama'u that these traditional remedies could also have such a strong effect on their love. The gifts of jewelry, clothes, and money were unmistakable displays of her boyfriend's devotion to her just as they were for Amira and Celine. Moreover, they gave him an excuse to admire her beauty and touch her.

Although Asama'u was initially fearful of visiting him in his room, this anxiety soon gave way:

> We continued to meet after my lessons. Then one day, he fell ill. When I told my friend, she advised me to visit him and bring him oranges. He was seriously sick. After that, I continued to check on him until he became well. I met him in his room and we chatted. Gradually, he seduced me into having sex. We watched American movies and I asked him questions about what the couples were doing, "Why is he touching and holding her?" and so on. And then, he would explain. So, things went on this way until I became totally infatuated with him and we had sex. I did not know what was happening. . . . I knew he was playing with my senses, telling me if I had sex with him, my relatives would allow us to marry. So with that in mind, I continued to sleep with him. I do not know what his thoughts were. I just knew I loved him and him me . . . so we continued with the relationship and I would tell my friend what we were doing. She would teach

me new things to do whenever I was with him. He used to give me pills every day, and when I left for [boarding] school, he bought me a term's supply.

Because few young women in Nigeria have had formal sex education in schools, much of what they learn about love, romance, and sex comes from family members, such as older sisters or cousins, friends, and boyfriends, or through books and television. As Asama'u narrated this experience, she described how her friend would coach her on how to care for her boyfriend. Her gift of oranges and careful attention demonstrated to him what a good girlfriend she was – and even what a good wife she could be. It also gave her another excuse to see him.

Although "blue films" (pornography) and foreign films with explicit sexual content are found across the country, people explained to me it is unusual for young men and women in northern Nigeria to watch these films together. Nevertheless, I often heard stories about married men who would show films to their new brides to teach them how to have sex. By asking her boyfriend questions about couples' sex scenes, Asama'u was potentially attempting to display her innocence and modesty to him. She may also have been "testing" him to see whether he was interested in having sex with her.

Even though Asama'u claimed her boyfriend seduced her into having sex, they both were willing to proceed. Her friend would exchange details with her about how to further convince him of her love. Although Asama'u emphasized that she was tricked into having sex the first time, she continued to have sex with him because she expected to marry him. She did not remember the name of the pills he gave her, but we both knew it was a form of contraception.

Asama'u continued:

My parents still insisted they did not want him to marry me. They sent me away for a few months. As soon as I got back, I went straight to his place, only to be met by a friend of his. He asked me, "Have you not been around? Your boyfriend has gotten married!" I could not believe it! So I went back home and cried. . . . Afterwards, he returned to me, proclaiming his love. But I no longer felt anything for him. I blamed him and my parents. But I do not blame myself. If my parents had let us marry, none of this would have happened . . . anyway, before we had separated, I had suitors I would never pay any attention to, so I simply moved on with one of them. Although this new boyfriend was no match for my first, I simply forgot my previous relationship and moved on. This time, I was wiser and did not love like before.

I did not understand how her boyfriend could marry another woman so quickly. When I discussed this with others, one woman explained to me that she was certain it was because he married either a former girlfriend or a girlfriend he courted while he was sleeping with Asama'u. During her stay with her relatives, my one friend ventured, her boyfriend most likely would have visited her house while she was away, especially if he remained sincere in his interest to marry her. Most men would want to find out details about when their girlfriends will return. This boyfriend might even have tried once again to convince her family members of his interest in marriage. With Asama'u out of town, her family could have taken that opportunity to threaten the boyfriend to stay away from her.

It is also possible, another of my key informants posited, that he was indeed playing with or "styling" her mind; that is, he fooled her into falling in love, aided by his potions. He may never have been sincere in his interest in marriage. The fact that he secretly gave her birth control pills made them suspicious. If a young woman gets pregnant out of wedlock, there is no question that it would be a shameful thing. However, many parents would consent to a marriage if they learned their daughter was pregnant.

Despite the fact that the boyfriend came back to convince Asama'u of his love, I think there is little chance he would have ended his current marriage. By saying she did not love like before, Asama'u meant that in future relationships she would feign love or interest, playing with men's senses instead of letting them play with hers. Although Asama'u claimed to "feel nothing," she undoubtedly was embarrassed by his rejection. By emphasizing how she did not blame herself, she may have been attempting to minimize her feelings of disappointment and vulnerability to me. Asama'u instead stressed that she directed her anger toward her parents. Her bitter tone reverberated through her narrative of her next two "serious" boyfriends. When she learned of her HIV test result a few years later, she blamed her positive status on the fact that her parents forbade this marriage.

AMIRA

As Amira told me about the first time she met John, I assumed she meant that a marriage would soon follow. I was surprised to learn later that she had a second boyfriend at the same time. She described, "I met another young guy who was very fair skinned. He was also tall and cute. Then, he was a degree student. So he just came around my school over his school's break . . . he came over and said he loved me! I turned to him and I said, 'Leave me alone! You are the whole talk of the school. Everybody is after you. So, I do not like you!' "

She continued,

> But then, he followed me to our house. I was quiet and did not speak to him. . . . He came back to the house later in the day. The security man [at the gate of our house] asked him who he was looking for. He met with my sister. She asked him, "Does she know you are coming?" He said no. She said, "I will go and get her for you." My sister went inside the house and called me, "Hey! Come outside and see a very 'big looking' [beautiful, rich man] for you outside . . . he speaks very good English and he was studying engineering or a science subject . . . besides, your other boyfriend [John] is not around. He has traveled. So nobody is going to tell him." So, she encouraged me to go. I went and he was so romantic – more than John!

"Like how?" I prompted with a smile.

> We sat at a bench outside our gate. My neighborhood was a quiet area, so I switched off the lights. He then came closer to me . . . later, he held my hands with his hands. He massaged them little by little. I was enjoying it. Later, he held me. Then next, it was my first kiss. When he kissed me, I felt so happy. I said, "God, wow!" I then felt John must not think I am attractive, since he could not kiss me or even touch me. I had one friend who would tell me that, if he likes you, he will make love to you, kiss you, romance you, hold you, touch you . . . but your current boyfriend [John] does not do this to you. He loves other girls and does this to them. He gives me gifts, but gifts are not love. . . . So when this guy, [Hassan], kissed me – my first kiss – I was so happy. He said, "Let us leave the area. Let us leave our gate." He held me around the waist. We were walking and gisting (chatting) just like a couple. Though he did not have anything to give me, he was so romantic. Just so, so romantic. . . . He said he liked my mouth. And he always talked about my dimple . . . and my smile. So when he said

such things, I would become so happy. As time went on, the love I had for John began to fade away. I only went to his place because of the gifts and the money.

I asked Amira if John ever found out. She explained that eventually he suspected that something was up. One afternoon, he returned home to Kano and went to collect her from school, only to see this other young man waiting for her. "When he saw us," Amira explained with a laugh, "he was so shocked. He was like, 'How?!'" and she made an impression of his aghast expression.

> John was shouting, just insulting the guy. It was the first time I heard him say that he wants to marry me. . . . He said, "I have been keeping her from men like you, who want to spoil her for me!" I felt so embarrassed. . . . I told John that he did not love me. Hassan is the guy that truly loves me. He kissed me. He touched me. He really loved me. So he was like, "What? I am away just two weeks, you already know all these things?" We were just fighting throughout the day. . . . Later that night, John came back to my house. I said, "What are you doing here?" He said I forgot my wristwatch in his car. He brought different kinds of fruits for my mother and me. He brought an apple, and that was the first time I ate an apple. He bought ice cream and then chocolates for me. Then for my mother, he bought a big can of powdered milk, and sugar with bread, and two cloth wrappers. . . . He bought cream-colored *sheda* [cloth] for my father. And then, he brought pairs of shoes for my mother and my father. Finally, he brought a chain and earrings in a case for me. . . . He was on his knees begging me, saying please, he is sorry. It is not that he does not love me. He felt if he tried "those things" with me, it would show he does not love me because I come from a Muslim home. I would think he is a bad person. . . . Then, he asked me if I did anything with the other guy. I asked, "Like what?" "Did he de-virgin you? Did he make love to you?" I said, "No." Then he said, "Promise me that you will not see him again." I said to him, "I love that guy. He is very handsome. I cannot say I will not ever see him again, but I promise you that I will not go to that extent."

I asked, "So what happened next?" Amira told me how John arranged their marriage:

> He told me that he wanted to go and see my mother and father. So I walked him to the house. He greeted my mother. Then, it was like "a man's world." They did the negotiating. He introduced himself to them for the first

time. . . . My parents had seen his gifts, but they had never met him face to face. So, John made his intention known to them – that he wanted to marry me as soon I finished my secondary education. So my parents said, "It is okay." They said, "You are welcome." My dad said that he likes his children to get married at young ages. So my father accepted him. . . . My mother said [the marriage] is okay, as long as he allowed me to practice my own religion [Islam]. Then John said, "Yes." The main reason why my father accepted him was because he was educated. He had his master's degree. My father asked John, "Are you going to send my daughter to school?" He said he would send me to university and even go further. That is the intention.

Amira explained to me that, in her family's tradition, if a man introduced himself to his girlfriend's family, made his marriage intentions known to her parents, and brought his own family to meet them, they considered him to be that woman's husband. She should then stop seeing her other boyfriends.

Amira was initially reluctant to do this. She returned to Hassan, and explained to him that the other man, John, was taking care of her far better than he could. He provided her money for books, uniforms, and school fees. At first, they tried to keep their relationship secret. Amira told him, "I love you, but one thing I want you to do is to please pretend as if nothing is going on. While he is away, if you are back from school, we can meet. But when he is around, we pretend as if nothing is happening." However, she eventually realized that it would be a long time before Hassan could save enough money to marry her. Amira knew a marriage was simply not possible, and her sister advised her to just marry John. She said that he could provide for her and she would be less of a burden on the family. Sadly, Amira ended the relationship with Hassan.

As illustrated in the cases above, some men may just be admirers – those who pass by women on the street or in school. Other women have boy-friends in different locations – one at home and the other at school or work. They would exchange phone numbers with these men and perhaps meet and chat once in a while. A woman may collect his gifts – such as credits for her cell phone, transportation money, or some food items – but not consider him her true love.

Boyfriends might also be more like friends and closer to women's own age. They may flirt with one another and even joke that they are husband

and wife. These men give women not only gifts but also attention and affection. Because there is less of an age difference between them, some women will feel less intimidated by their advances. They are more likely to touch, kiss, or even sleep with these boyfriends. However, because of their age, they often do not have the wealth nor perhaps the inclination to seriously consider marriage. Women, therefore, might continue to see them from time to time, but they must wait to see how these men mature before making a commitment. Amira hoped that Hassan could eventually support her in the way her future husband, John, currently does, but it became increasingly unlikely that he would be able to do so.

Still, older, wealthy men eagerly seek relationships with young women, like Amira. These men are often able to provide poor women and their families with expensive gifts, including both subsistence goods, such as groceries, and consumer items, such as clothes, handbags, and shoes. They may offer to pay the school fees for their girlfriends or, if the women are older, money to start shops or other businesses if they want to work. Even if a woman comes from a relatively privileged background, I was told that she might still ask her boyfriend for assistance with a pressing need early in the courtship. In this case, she is testing the man to see if he is stingy with his money.

Older men are also able to draw upon their maturity to provide women advice on their education and career goals, family concerns, or other issues. Men take a great deal of pride in their ability to counsel others. Likewise, when women discuss what they like most about their partners, they often cite men's wisdom and guidance. Older boyfriends, they explained to me, already had success in their education and careers, and they hope to learn from their experiences.

Although women know that some of these suitors are only looking for pretty, young women to impress their peers, others may be potential marriage partners. Again, women are careful to keep these boyfriends from knowing that other men are pursuing them. They fear that if a man finds out about her other boyfriends, he could threaten them – or her – with violence or take revenge in other ways. Amira witnessed this response firsthand in a confrontation between John and Hassan. Since John knew she still had feelings for Hassan, Amira would sabotage her marriage plans if she continued her relationship with him. Because this secret was exposed, she yielded. This, however, was not Amira's last relationship before her marriage.

MR. LECTURER

Soon after Amira ended the relationship with Hassan, John was transferred to Lagos. She recently began a postsecondary school certificate program in biology, and he provided her a car to take her back and forth from school. There, Amira met her third serious boyfriend. She was talking with her friends outside of the classroom when one of her lecturers called her into his office. He said that he liked her and implied his interest in sleeping with her. He then threatened that she better not turn him down. Amira said to me she had never slept with a man before and was unsure what to do. She told him she would think it over and left. Amira went back to her friends for advice. They told her that if she wanted to pass the class, she must say yes to him. I asked Amira how her friends knew this, and she said that they told her about another classmate, who he also approached. This young woman refused him and he failed her. Because John wanted her to study hard and pass the class, Amira felt that she had to say yes. And, since he was not in Kano, she knew that he would not find out about it. Although Amira was afraid, she told the lecturer, "It is okay."

The lecturer then began to meet Amira after classes and they would visit different romantic sites around the campus and city. Shortly thereafter, they slept together. I asked Amira if she thought he had genuine feelings for her and she immediately said no, but he claimed to love her. She again described the assorted gifts he bought her. First, it was handbags. Amira added, "So when my husband gave me money for handbags, I would save the money." Then, he gave her a phone, which she gave away to her brother. She summarized her conflicted feelings, "It was like, my husband was thinking that he was the one that was sponsoring my education, but it was the lecturer." At the end of her first year, the school named her the top student in her program. Amira knew this man was responsible for her ranking.

Amira said she was not happy with her relationship with the lecturer. She also knew she had to keep it secret from John. He took her to a doctor, who gave her an injection every few months to prevent pregnancy. Although her parents were not aware of the injections, Amira said she did tell them about their relationship. According to her, they too agreed that there was nothing they could do. Her parents were afraid that if she failed, John would then go to the school to find out why she was doing so poorly. He would hear about the lecturer and call off the wedding, they thought. While all Nigerians would condemn this behavior as immoral and unacceptable, lecturers have tremendous influence over their students.

Amira explained,

> So that was how it went on. My lecturer did not want to see me with any other man. Whenever other students made advances toward me, he would trace them and fail them. So I became very, very famous because of my lecturer. Everyone knew about us . . . I would go to the school cafeteria with friends and eat anything I liked for free. He would go and pay the bill. He spent a lot of money on me. As time went on, he knew my home. He knew my family was not doing well. He bought three, four, five bags of rice to distribute to us.

I asked Amira if he was legitimate competition with John, and she quickly dismissed that thought. He was much too old for her, she said. In addition, he was married to another lecturer at a nearby university and they had children. Although he appeared to be sincere in his intention to marry her as his second wife, Amira reiterated to me again how scared she was of him. She explained that he was a Nupe man from Niger State and that Nupe people were very wicked. "They charm people and destroy their lives," Amira stressed.

When John was transferred back to Kano, Amira said that she confessed everything to him. According to her, he too feared what would happen to her education if she rejected the lecturer, so he was reluctant to intervene. Instead, he hastened their wedding plans. Against the advice of her parents, Amira was baptized in his church, and they sought religious counseling in preparation for the marriage.

Then, the lecturer heard a rumor about the wedding. When he called her, Amira reminded him of her engagement to another man. She added, "I am too young for you. You are fifty and I am almost age-mates with some of your children." When the lecturer dismissed Amira's explanation and expressed his own plan to marry her, she replied, "*Gaskiya* (Honestly), truly, sincerely speaking, I do not want to get married to you. I like my husband. I told him that I have a high enough GPA. Even if I leave him, nothing will happen to me."

The lecturer was furious. As their final exams approached, Amira went to the exam officer to tell her that she feared the lecturer would attempt to fail her. All of the faculty in the department knew about the affair and did not like it. They hesitated to intervene, however, because Amira had consented to it. Sure enough, the lecturer did attempt to fail her by changing the time of the exams. She was alerted just before the exam took place. Because it was ecology, a subject she found easy, she finished the paper very quickly and then went outside to wait.

While the rest of the students were inside the classroom completing their exams, the lecturer stormed in to see if she was there. The officer told him that she had already finished it. Amira said her classmates told her that the lecturer then fell down on the floor, crying and shouting. He claimed that the exam was canceled. He told the room that she was a prostitute and cheated on the test.

The department administrators take accusations of exam malpractice very seriously, Amira said. The dean thus summoned her to give her testimony. She told the dean everything that the lecturer purchased for her: a generator, furniture, gas, clothing, gifts, and money – "probably worth over a million naira [~$7,000]!" she claimed. John also attended this meeting.

Amira said that she had never loved the lecturer. She pretended she had feelings for him because she feared failing out of school. After investigating the issue, the dean accepted that she did not cheat, but still she was awarded a grade of E, which meant she would have to retake the class. The lecturer, however, was demoted. They reduced his salary and changed his office. "The case was so famous in the school!" Amira proclaimed.

The mythical qualities of this story were hard for me to ignore. I was suspicious about the details. Did the lecturer really throw a hysterical fit in the middle of the lecture hall? Did Amira actually fear he would threaten her life with a spiritual curse if she rejected him? And, why would Amira's parents and fiancé remain silent when they learned that she was in a relationship with her lecturer? Did she really tell them she was having sex with him?

Despite some of the likely exaggerations and holes in Amira's narrative, there are still important social facts to be discerned from it. Most prominently, her description of the affair reveals how women often depend on men to access educational opportunities. In northern Nigeria, men dominate occupations in both the formal and informal economy. As women begin to access higher education, they are raised with the idea that their schooling will allow them to acquire resources previously available only to a few of the most elite women in the north: jobs with an income, savings, and economic autonomy. They can assist their families and marry educated men who share these values. Women ultimately aspire to gain greater power in their relationships with men through education. They hope that their husbands will respect their decisions, listen to their reasoning, and consider the advice they offer them.

These educational aspirations are dominant themes across women's narratives of their first loves – held both by parents and young women. Many fear that their relationships with men will rob them of these opportunities because of the effort and time that wives must devote to caring for their families. And yet – as Amira's narrative clearly reveals – intimate relationships may also provide them with the resources they need to pursue these goals, while also helping to support women and their families. Boyfriends or husbands "sponsor" women's higher education by paying their school fees. Women may also be tempted into relationships with men in order to pass their classes. These economic inequalities thus reproduce social inequalities, where men are able to maintain their power and control over women through these exchanges.

Although Amira was unhappy with this sexual relationship, her jubilant expression at the end of her story illuminated the pride she felt in having exacted what she needed from the lecturer and triumphed. At no point in her narrative did Amira present herself as a passive victim. Indeed, she used the gifts and money this man gave her to support her family. They also allowed Amira to become popular on campus and fend off advances from other men who knew they had no chance. Her high grades and rankings in her program motivated her to continue her education. At the very end of her story, when she learned she would have to repeat the course, Amira explained that she felt encouraged to study even harder to prove to the department that she did not need the assistance of this lecturer. In fact, Amira said, she aspired to become a lecturer herself in the future.

Finally, her lecturer's demotion demonstrated to Amira that she had the ability to not just subvert but actually overturn these power structures that coerce women like her into undesirable sexual relationships. Amira did not seek to reject these dominating relationships altogether, however. Rather, she did not want to disappoint her future husband by failing out of school. Amira's education was symbolic of her virtue as a new bride in a prosperous, respectable, and modern marriage.

LOVE LIVES

The women in this chapter, I argue, are part of a generation of young northern Nigerian women who have been exposed to a new set of opportunities alongside unyielding social constraints. Although they are not wealthy, many young women's families now expect them to receive a Western education, in addition to religious schooling. However, there are few prospects for salaried positions upon the completion of their diplomas, certificates, and degrees. Furthermore, school fees and expenses often remain beyond the reach of poor families, prohibiting young women from finishing secondary school or university. Thus, women frequently continue to remain dependent on men for financial support, social status, and wisdom. Even as political and economic forces have conspired to strip youth of the social privileges that the completion of education and formal employment should provide, this generation of women is nonetheless committed to fashioning identities, families, and life trajectories distinct from the times of their parents' marriages. Their socioeconomic aspirations, I observed, are enmeshed in intimate relationships.

Regardless of religion or ethnicity, the young women in this chapter desired love-based relationships not arranged marriages. What makes these romantic exploits unique from generations before them, arguably, is how women materially experience intimacy–namely, through the gifts they receive from their boyfriends. When a man clasps a necklace around a woman's neck and praises her beauty, for example, she feels a surge of pleasure. However, in the case of these particular young women, gifts do not necessarily come from a single person. As I show, different kinds of exchanges take place with different partners. Like their male counterparts, women may have numerous boyfriends at the same time: a few admirers, a companion, a guy who is not "serious" but likes to have fun, and still others who are wealthy and much older.

Through these exchanges, women attempt to gain access to financial wealth, social privilege, and maturity. These gifts are not just offered to individual women; they are also directed to women's family members. While some receive handbags and cell phones from one boyfriend, they may also receive food or money from another, which they then share. Whether luxurious commodities or subsistence goods, gifts exist within a larger moral economy in which these objects not only highlight prosperity and generosity but also symbolize women's desirability and respectability. Even so, such exchanges solidify and reproduce the systems of inequalities that subordinate women to their boyfriends and their families. And finally, sex is not just an outcome of a couple's growing intimacy. It also serves as an object of exchange from women to men, as they navigate and invest in this web of dependencies.

How, then, do women attempt to assert their agency and secure power in their relationships given these competing pressures and limitations? As I point out, one of the defining features in these four women's narratives is the conspicuous presentation of some features of their relationships – and their discretion over others. Women strategically use speech – and silence – to convey their interest to certain men while deflecting the interest of others. A woman's refusal to speak to an admirer might actually communicate her openness to a relationship, which Celine demonstrated.

Likewise, a woman's ability to speak evasively and not immediately reject an admirer, even if she is uninterested, may prolong a relationship in which she collects gifts in exchange for her occasional attention, as Patience described. Women may then disguise the fact that they redistribute these gifts to their parents, siblings, or friends. Young women work to display their beauty, status, and virtue while hiding the fact that they may come from poor families.

Even in sexual relationships, women are careful in their self-presentation efforts, which center on protecting their dignity. This was especially clear in the way Asama'u attempted to subtly intimate her innocence to her boyfriend by asking him about couples' sexual activities in films. Both

Asama'u and Amira were given "hidden" forms of family planning by their respective partners of which they could also claim ignorance because people receive injections and medications for an array of concerns. The couple may then continue a sexual relationship within this face-saving realm of ambiguity. Such measures stand in contrast to other modes of contraception, such as condoms, which are visible symbols of this knowledge, premarital or extramarital sexual experience, and, consequently, widely acknowledged as immoral.

While these acts of concealment and exposure may indeed reflect women's exercise of agency, they are also implicated in their heightened risk of contracting HIV. As young, unmarried women bear the brunt of politicians' and religious leaders' accusations of immorality – and a faithful, monogamous marriage is promoted as the solution to HIV prevention – married women, until recently, have been largely overlooked as vulnerable to the virus. Next, I will focus on the set of social and economic constraints and acts of intimate violence that shape married women's exposure to HIV and the ways they cope in the aftermath of their diagnosis.

2

_____ ❧ _____

Twice Married

Jummai was fifteen years old when she met the man she would eventually marry. Born in northern Nigeria, she spent her childhood in
Cameroon. A mutual friend shared his photograph with Jummai, and she
sent her picture to him in return. "Really," she said, "at the time, I just wanted
to see if he had any 'defects,' and then I would say yes. I always wanted to
marry someone from far away." This man traveled frequently to her city on
business. When he first called on her, she liked him immediately. Jummai
then introduced her boyfriend to her family. Next, he returned with his
parents to ask Jummai's parents for their approval. They consented to
the marriage. His family presented them with an offering of kola nuts as
a sign of their gratitude. After two months, they came back to Jummai's
home with a suitcase filled with cloth. His family gave these items to her
relatives to announce the engagement. They set the wedding date. Soon
after that, they brought Jummai's *kayan lefe* (the groom's gift to the bride).

As she described her wedding ceremony to me, Jummai's face lit up:

> During the wedding, my husband stayed with friends in my town. In our
> culture, the bride hides on the night of the "bride catching," which is also
> called *kamu*. The groom's parents come in search of her and "bargain"
> with her friends for her release from the room. The bride is then brought
> out crying. Next, the ceremonies started and they applied henna to my
> skin. My fiancé's parents came and bathed me in perfume. They dressed
> me in new clothes and pampered me with cosmetics. They then "sprayed"
> money on me (placed small bills on her head to show their appreciation,

often while dancing around her). . . . New brides are usually taken to their mothers' rooms for advice, scolding, and preaching in preparation for married life. My mother advised me to do everything my husband said I should do. This advice went on for hours until *Maghrib* (evening) prayers, when elderly women took me to my husband's house.

While all of this was happening inside Jummai's home, her husband's friends came with cars to pick up a "fake bride" – one of her friends – after paying a sum of money. They drove around the town singing and celebrating. Jummai's husband did not return until the morning after the ceremony. This time, her friends were present and playfully paid money for "the coming of the groom." Jummai was terrified of what was going to happen after her friends left, she recounted. "I had never left my home before and now I was alone with a man!" Reflecting on this moment, she summarized, "It was a new life and I did not know how it would unfold."

In northern Nigeria, marriage initiates a critical transformation in a woman's social role from that of a child into that of an adult. The relative freedom of women to select – and ignore – suitors is a recent phenomenon. Older generations had little choice in their marital partners.[1] While these attitudes have changed somewhat over the past decades, marriage remains practically compulsory. Women almost always secure the permission of their families before they wed. Nigerians widely acknowledge marriage as a mechanism for whole families to achieve upward social mobility. Introductions, matchmaking, and formally arranged marriages reflect families' efforts to extend economic support to young women.

Marriage is not merely a religious obligation; couples must marry for families to expand. Northern Nigerian women give birth, on average, to six or more children over the course of their lives. Marriage also precipitates the reproduction of cultural traditions, social status, and power relations. The moral and cultural foundations that shape the formation of families, such as marriage and childbirth, justify particular imbalances of power in northern Nigerian society. These include elders' control over the young, and men over women.[2]

Contemporary marriages in Nigeria take place in a political and economic context where many men and women are underemployed or unemployed. Men may feel overwhelmed by debt or pressured by unrelenting pleas for support from relatives. Their inconsistent incomes limit their ability to meet these expectations. They cannot adequately save the resources they need to provide for large families. Facing these emasculating economic constraints, young and old men may attempt to imitate their wealthy peers by courting girlfriends and marrying new wives. Extramarital relationships allow men to uphold their sexual reputations.[3] They seek remarriage, despite their inability to afford weddings. Women feel powerless in their efforts to prevent husbands from pursuing girlfriends and polygamous marriages. Although women's extramarital relationships are less common, many of my key informants remained in contact with past boyfriends and admirers. They also do not necessarily decline gifts of money or other tokens, if offered.[4]

While marriage may be obligatory, marital relationships are often quite fragile. Demographers report that Hausa Muslim communities' divorce rates rank among the highest in the world.[5] A man may divorce his wife a single time and then reconcile soon after. When he states his desire to divorce three times out loud, he terminates the possibility of reconciliation – this statement is called *talaka*. While divorce is less common among Christians, men may still invest their resources in other relationships and abandon their wives. This, in effect, ends a marriage without a formal divorce. Given the sometimes substantial age differences between marital partners, husbands may widow their wives well before their reproductive years conclude. While widows feel somewhat less pressure to remarry than divorcees, women of reproductive age usually intend to marry again.[6]

When faced with the threat of marital dissolution, women fear calling attention to instances of abuse, infidelity, and neglect. If they disclose these violations, their families may ignore, dismiss, or downplay their complaints. Civil or religious courts may not protect them, unless they also have supportive family members and sufficient economic resources. Moreover, both families and courts will encourage reconciliation over dissolution. If a husband ends the marriage, he can take custody of their children, evict his wife from the house, and even seize her possessions. This often happens with few or no sanctions.[7] A divorce rarely provides a clear-cut termination of a relationship. Rather, it produces a morass of unfulfilled or partially fulfilled claims. These social ties, obligations, and dependencies shape women's experiences as they proceed from one marriage to the next.

While men engage in extramarital relationships and women circulate through husbands, these movements create the epidemiological conditions through which HIV is transmitted within marriage in northern Nigeria.[8] The virus is enmeshed in complex emotional experiences, embodied forms of suffering, economic instability, and interpersonal conflicts between husbands and wives. All of these social forces profoundly affect women's lives as they cope with hardships related to their newly diagnosed illness. This deeply stigmatizing diagnosis exposes taken-for-granted assumptions about faith, family, the home, intimacy, and the body. Such tacit beliefs materialize often because public misperceptions about HIV suggest women have violated moral principles in their domestic lives.

At the center of these negotiations, the question of secrecy resurfaces: men and women may hide not only their HIV status but also past or current extramarital relationships, instances of abuse, and debts, among others. Many women commit to keeping their husbands' secrets – including both ordinary and earth-shattering betrayals – even when their husbands refuse to do the same. Women guard this knowledge to salvage power and protect their well-being. And yet, by doing so, they often remain silent over, and even defend, men's dominant and dominating privileges. They give far more than they receive in sometimes futile attempts to safeguard their reputations.

Although this chapter documents themes common in many northern Nigerian marriages, I intend to focus here on the singularity of two women's experiences. Jummai and Mairo confront devastating betrayals in their relationships that dislodge their expectation that marriage can offer them a moral, social, and economic refuge. They grapple with the ethical question: what should women do when they possess knowledge of their husbands' duplicitous acts? In their first marriages, they both face being discredited because of infertility and domestic abuse – not issues related specifically to HIV. While Jummai opts to hide her first husband's deeply stigmatized condition, Mairo broadcasts her husband's maltreatment of her to the public. When these marriages ended – Jummai was widowed and Mairo divorced – their respective experiences contoured the trajectories of their subsequent relationships. Furthermore, they shape the circumstances through which they contracted HIV.

JUMMAI

The anticipation, joy, and fears that Jummai felt in her *amarya* (recent bride) life quickly gave way to frustration and concern. After four years of marriage, Jummai and her husband had yet to conceive a baby. She elaborated: "We discussed the issue of children, birth, and fertility almost every day! . . . We sought medical advice, went for tests, took drugs, and received lots of guidance, including prayers. I never conceived . . . When he told me he intended to remarry, I did not feel bad. I thought that I was the cause of the problem."

A successful childbirth in northern Nigeria confirms a woman's status as an adult and fulfills her primary obligation to her husband. Men, in turn, acquire authority both in the household and in the larger patrilineage. Nigerians view parenthood as the most sacred responsibility of married adults and a form of social insurance. As people age, they hope their children will care for them. No one wants to die alone, women repeatedly stressed. Parents inculcate beliefs about elders' power and moral authority in their children to secure their own support in old age. Consequently, couples endure powerful feelings of distress when they experience infertility. It disrupts processes of social reproduction and further aggravates already uneven power relations between men and women.[9]

Nigeria, like many other countries characterized by high fertility rates, reports concurrently high rates of infertility. Despite the fact that men account for at least half of all instances of infertility and couples suffer the consequences of childlessness together, families commonly fault women for these reproductive failures. In Islamic Hausa tradition, a wife's infertility usually motivates a husband to marry additional wives. It also serves as a ground for the marriage's dissolution. The conflicts that transpire from infertility produce intense anxiety, frustration, and sadness, especially among women. An infertile woman's family and community may ostracize her. And, given this stigma, many Nigerians assert that it is unlikely that a woman known to be infertile can find a desirable husband.[10]

Over the first five years of their marriage, Jummai reluctantly but courageously accepted the blame for her husband's infertility, assuming it was her fault. She anticipated he would eventually divorce her. Instead, he married a second wife. There are a number of reasons that could account for his decision to do so. If a man marries an infertile wife, his family will pressure him to find another wife who can bear children. If her husband refused, they would have raised concerns about the nature of their marriage and, specifically, Jummai's character. They would speculate on the measures she took to stop her husband from remarrying.

Northern Nigerian films and novels, for example, frequently feature women who seek the advice of *mallams* to keep their husbands from marrying again. No one I knew would admit to obtaining these charms, but I am sure they possessed them. Women carefully guard knowledge of these mystical objects and their purposes from others. Nigerians, nevertheless, generally believe that women's efforts to prevent these relationships from forming are unacceptable, even if they are common. They say that such women have too much power over men.

Jummai later learned that her husband had hidden from her – and from his new bride – the laboratory test results confirming he was the source of their reproductive challenges. Because of this information, he did not possess religious grounds for dissolving their marriage, Jummai explained. However, this would not stop many northern Muslim men from proceeding with divorce. I got the sense from Jummai that they also felt genuine affection for each other. Perhaps her husband's guilt or fear of exposure motivated him to treat his wives more kindly. Even so, he risked jeopardizing his reputation if he did not remarry. His peers would ridicule him because he lacked children. Although communities and families subject men to far less stigma than women for the same condition, Jummai's husband would still have difficulty finding another spouse. He thus went to great lengths to cover his secret.[11]

Unsurprisingly, his second wife did not get pregnant either. Jummai then felt sure her husband was the cause of their infertility. She also learned that she was not his first wife. He had married and divorced a wife prior to her. His former wife, Jummai heard, could not cope with the marriage. This, she speculated, was related to their inability to have children, although she had no proof. Just like Jummai, his new wife also remained resolute in her commitment to the marriage. They conspired to keep his condition secret, and their families instead faulted them for their infertility, not their husband. Jummai and her co-wife remained married to their husband until he died almost fifteen years later.

Given the country's high rates of marital dissolutions, a childless marriage that lasts fifteen years is, in fact, quite unusual. It raises the following questions: Why did Jummai and her co-wife live with their husband for such a long period? Why protect their husband's secret and shoulder the stigma of infertility in the eyes of their community? In short, why endure so much – suffering their husband's illness on his behalf – just to protect his reputation? Jummai and her co-wife vigorously defended the same patriarchal values that northern Nigerian men so frequently deploy to strip women of their power and security in relationships. One answer for this lies in the fact that wives usually needs their husbands' consent to dissolve marriages. Jummai's husband may have resisted giving them his permission for a divorce because he feared people would learn his secret. Whether true or not, I do not think this point explains the entire story.

Jummai emphasized that her commitment to the marriage displayed her virtuous character. She believed that the care and support she offered her husband affirmed her standing as a respectable wife even amid widespread suspicion that she was infertile. Judging by the tone of our discussion, I got the impression that Jummai felt quite secure in this marriage. Perhaps her knowledge of her husband's vulnerability meant that he would not hastily dispose of her for another wife. Infertility, in other words, may have produced a more intimate marriage, secured by their mutual efforts to protect each other's secrets.

Women, I argue, enter a "patriarchal bargain" when they choose to keep their husbands' secrets hidden. They commit to protecting a dominant notion of masculine power, which – on the surface – appears to work against their efforts to secure greater control in their relationships.[12] Jummai's efforts to conceal her husband's secret must be understood in a social context in which women also collude in keeping their own secrets from men. This carefully guarded knowledge allows them to protect their autonomy and preserve social ties with others. Indeed, in their interpretation of Islamic doctrine, women widely relate discretion with virtue. Northern Nigerian Muslims stress that if God desires people's secrets to be exposed, they cannot intervene in this divine plan. Many Muslim women understand this injunction to mean that they should not expose the contents of their own or others' secrets. Only God possesses that power.[13]

While women's decisions may focus on domestic responsibilities, their choice to protect their husbands' secrets cannot be fully appreciated without also questioning the larger social structures that orient their ethical sensibilities and reinforce uneven gendered power relations. Jummai's second marriage elucidates both the tolls that secrets take on women's bodies and – when secrets are exposed – the effects they have on their social relationships.

Following the death of her husband, Jummai returned to Kano from Cameroon. A man approached her with an interest in marriage. He already had three wives and recently paid a brideprice for a fourth when he met Jummai. Islam prohibits men from marrying more than four wives. Yet, as women point out, husbands circumvent this prohibition by divorcing one of these wives to marry a fifth. Jummai knew about this man's engagement, but she did not expect him to divorce his wife on her behalf. Nearly two years later, this man told her he ended his most recent marriage. He then proposed to her. In addition to his three current wives and the wife he recently divorced, her husband had been married two other times. Jummai was, in fact, his seventh bride.

Widows from childless marriages, like Jummai, encounter a great deal of stigma as they seek to remarry. Even if Jummai explained to prospective suitors about her first husband's infertility – and I am sure she tried – it would still raise suspicions. As part of the engagement process, families investigate the couple's respective backgrounds. They evaluate the social, economic, and reproductive histories of both the bride and groom. Her new fiancé's reputation as a womanizer and the capricious way in which he dissolved his former marriages unquestionably disconcerted Jummai. Furthermore, her concerns over his character were compounded by another fear: the poor condition of his health. Jummai described:

> At around the time of our wedding, I went to Sokoto Hospital because I had heard about HIV. I wanted to know my status. They told me I was negative . . . I even went for another confirmatory test and was negative still. I was thrilled, but I could not ask my fiancé to take a test. Even before our marriage, he was constantly ill. Sometimes, he would turn so dark. When I asked him about it, he would say he had piles (hemorrhoids). I was

afraid he would say I did not trust him if I requested him to go for a test.
Then, he would refuse to marry me. I was under pressure from my family
to get married because I lived at home and had not found another suitable
boyfriend. I also wanted to have my own home.

Jummai claimed she did not know whether HIV caused her husband's
illnesses. She also admitted she distrusted him. Even so, she needed to
remarry. When Jummai moved into his house, she learned two of his wives
constantly fell sick. He had rashes on his leg, which, he said, "must have
been something from the bush." His second wife had a persistent cold
and diarrhea, Jummai described. The third wife had problems with body
aches and fevers. Jummai said that she did not want to think about HIV.
She claimed she did not know all of the symptoms then and she did not
realize that she too could be infected with the virus.

More likely, I suspect, she did not want to create a conflict in the house
that might result in her divorce. After seven months of marriage, her
husband fell gravely ill. He stopped working. Jummai and the other wives
questioned the source of his sickness: "What type of illness does not respond to medications?" He said people cursed him because they did not
want to pay back their debts to him. Unknown to the wives at that time,
his brothers took him for an HIV test. Fully aware of their brother's status,
the family called the wives together to discuss the sickness. Then, they lied
to them and attributed his symptoms to anemia. The doctors needed to
screen their blood to see who could donate to him. Although the hospital
did not inform them of their results, they all tested positive. Soon after
this screening, the third wife passed away.

Jummai felt confused and misled by her husband and his family.
While she said that the wives worried about their husband's health,
in retrospect, I realized Jummai knew much more than she said to me.
She suspected he suffered from a disease shared between a man and his
partners. She knew his symptoms included rashes, fevers, and diarrhea.
The very fact that she sought a test before her marriage suggests she recognized the possibility of HIV. Although Nigerians have had access to
free, anonymous HIV counseling and testing at sites across the country
for well over a decade, people rarely seek a test out of curiosity alone.
Women generally receive screening for HIV after they fall sick or when
they go to hospitals for prenatal care.

Jummai was not so much in denial about HIV as she was acutely aware of the social repercussions its transmission would raise. For example, if she told one of her co-wives she suspected she had the virus, that wife might inform their husband. They would almost certainly blame Jummai. After spending fifteen years in her first marriage where she carefully hid her husband's infertile condition, she knew the possible consequences of exposing these closely guarded secrets.

Jummai continued:

> I tried to get the truth from him, but he would not give in and tell me. I would talk about different sexually transmitted diseases and other sicknesses going around these days . . . I even showed him my negative test results. He would say that I was too inquisitive: "What would you have done if you discovered I was positive at the time?" And I said, "I would not have married!"

Jummai's previous marriage taught her she could gain stability and perhaps even greater intimacy if she bore the burden of her husband's medical condition. I think her past experience informed her attempts to cajole her current husband into disclosing his status. By telling him about "different sexually transmitted diseases and other sicknesses going around," she hoped to open a window through which he could confide in her. In fact, she even gave him the opportunity to lie and name a cause other than HIV. Evidently, her former husband had no difficulty lying about his affliction. By showing her ability to forgive, she displayed her commitment to her marriage.

However, as Jummai's current husband resisted her efforts, she attempted a different tactic. Possibly thinking he refused to disclose because he blamed her for HIV, she shared the negative test result with him. By showing this document, she also indirectly threatened to reveal she knew what was *really* wrong. He brushed off her warning with an accusation of being "too inquisitive." This thinly veiled criticism implied she was not acting like a dutiful, modest wife.

By questioning what she would have done if she discovered he was positive at the time of their wedding, her husband sought to antagonize her. He obliquely intimated that he knew she needed to marry him. The circumstances surrounding her previous marriage limited her options.

By arguing back, "I would not have married!" Jummai attempted to save face. She did, in fact, marry him while suspecting he had the virus.

I asked Jummai whether the other wives also confronted their husband. She replied, "I was the only one who talked about it. The others never did. After some time, his brothers then gathered us and said he had TB [tuberculosis]. So, I asked if it was detectible in one's blood. And they said yes. Then, I asked if we had caught it. They said it was very possible. But, they said, we would not start treatment until our husband had finished taking his medications."

Jummai knew about the association between HIV and tuberculosis and the fact that diagnostic tests locate the virus in the blood. She again pleaded with her husband's brothers to acknowledge that he had passed his illness on to her. Even though they admitted the possibility of transmission, they refused to provide the wives' medications. Any doctor would have urged HIV-positive patients to bring their family members to the hospital for diagnosis and treatment. Clearly, they did not make this plan in consultation with the husband's physician. More likely, they did not want her or her co-wives to go to the clinic because then they would learn their status.

Jummai's husband finally divorced her. After he pronounced *talaka* ("I divorce you") three times, thereby shuttering the possibility of reconciliation, Jummai insisted he tell her his ailment. Her husband said to her, "That is why I have divorced you – in order to cleanse myself of any responsibility or blame for the infection – because you are my fourth and most recent wife." He then admitted to being HIV positive. When he could no longer hide his HIV status from his family or neighbors, her husband needed to accuse someone.

Anticipating divorce all along, Jummai reminded him of her proof that she was HIV negative at the time of marriage. She publicly accepted the fact that she was the source of their infection – again suffering her husband's illness on his behalf. In exchange, she demanded he acknowledge the truth to her. Although he told no one else, her husband conceded this point. He promised to provide her with money for her medical care and transportation to the hospital in exchange for her silence. Four months after this confession, he died.

Jummai's case illustrates the centrality of secrets in women's pursuit of power, support, and dignity in their marriages. However, she also revealed the consequences women face as a result of their complicity. In Jummai's case, her tacit agreement to hide her husband's condition denied her the possibility of having children over a fifteen-year period. And this, in turn, affected the course of her second marriage. While she distrusted her second husband, Jummai hoped that if he confided his diagnosis with her, the relationship would strengthen. And yet, as her desperation for his disclosure grew, he ultimately and unsurprisingly divorced her. Another bargain unfolded at the end of the marriage: she would not openly challenge his explanation for the divorce and, in return, he privately acknowledged that she did not infect the family. Once again, she suffered from her husband's illness – HIV infection – in exchange for the possibility of a stable, supportive marriage, which never ultimately materialized.

MAIRO

Mairo was in her late twenties when we first met. She grew up in the city of Kano. Like Jummai, she was married twice before. I began our interview by asking her to tell me about the time she met her first husband. Mairo said that her stepfather introduced them. This man complained that his current wife did not properly care for him. Mairo's stepfather told him he had a daughter. Taking pity on him, he encouraged this man to meet with her to see if she would be a suitable bride. They arranged the visit. Mairo knew that she did not like him, but she lied to her family about her feelings. Her stepfather asked her multiple times whether she genuinely loved him. Mairo insisted that she did. When I asked her why, she said, "I was afraid that if I said no, I would run into problems with both my parents and even my grandmother! I also agreed to marry him because my mother had advised me that you should not always say everything you think. Some things, you must simply swallow."

Mairo did not want her mother to think she disrespected her stepfather, nor did she want to insult him. In Kano, many families no longer formally force their daughters into marriages, but they continue to place considerable pressure on them to marry men they select. Mairo accepted the proposal.

I asked Mairo to tell me about her wedding and her life as an *amarya*. She began:

The date for the wedding was fixed. Then, we were married. My friends were so happy. After I was taken to my husband's house, I spent a week ignoring him. Even when he spoke to me, I refused to answer. I was always in a bad mood. He would corner me and force me to have sex. I kept running away to my parents' home, only to be sent back to him. So, even though we continued to have sex, I was very cold and unapproachable. He had to leave my money for food on the table because I refused to speak to him. After four months of this attitude, he started to beat me. Sometimes he would beat me severely and then proceed to have sex with me. But sometimes, he would not succeed, as I would even bite him!

Regardless of their feelings about marriage, the women I interviewed almost always stressed the terror, shame, and powerlessness they felt as their families lured them into the bedroom to meet their new husbands and have sex for the first time. Women told me about how they ran away or resisted their husbands' attempts to sleep with them. They recalled excruciating pain and described the blood they often saw on their bedsheets the next morning.

Although these were unquestionably frightening experiences for many women, Hausa society circulates similar narratives about the importance of virginity and virtuous brides. Men and their families expect wives to possess modest dispositions. If a young woman lacks *kunya* (shame) or even appears to enjoy having sex, her husband might suspect that his new bride has had previous sexual partners. Traditionally, a Muslim family inspects bed linens for drops of blood, which indicate the bride's purity. Women take a great deal of pride in their status as virgin brides.

Mairo provided a far more detailed and violent account than most other women I met. She barely paused to mention the wedding itself. Her friends may have been happy at the wedding reception, but she felt no pleasure or pride. Many northern Nigerians would say that Mairo acted dishonorably in her deliberate effort to ignore her new husband. They expect brides to demonstrate courteous, deferential, and obedient behavior. Mairo was aloof and defiant. She felt humiliated when she tried to explain to her family why she needed to leave his house, only to be sent back to him. Her protests, in other words, fell on deaf ears.

Women hesitate to report acts of domestic violence to their families, much less the police. They fear if the police apprehend their husbands, they will lose their means of support. Their husbands will end the marriage. Spouses may also intensify their abuse if their wives file complaints. Legislative attempts to criminalize domestic violence and protect the rights of victims at the national level have made advances only in recent years. Few women I met knew about these legal protections or made use of them.

Given women's reluctance to report domestic violence to their families, Mairo's case is again unusual. She continued:

> Finally, after some time, my stepfather intervened and told my husband that he did not give me to him to be beaten. My husband promised not to beat me again. My stepfather told him to document it. The next time I am beaten, the marriage is over. But then, not long after, his first wife came to my house and asked if we were around. They had fought. She came looking to fight with me, but I was not home. When I came back, my husband was there and he was seething with anger. I asked him for money for food and he said there was no money. I was cooking rice and it had started to boil, so I took it off the stove (to deny him his dinner). He asked me why I did this. He then began insulting my parents, so I prepared myself and tied my scarf around my waist. I returned every insult he threw at me, telling him, "Not my parents!" He then beat me thoroughly. I was crying out to God to save me. I said, "Oh my God, divorce me," until I could no longer speak. He punched me in the jaw and nose that night, and then he left me alone in the house. While all this was happening, our neighbors came out and begged him to unlock the door. But he would not listen to them. The next morning, I went outside the house and headed for the toilet. My neighbor saw me and advised me not to leave him. I told her no. She said to go on and have my bath, massage my body, and take some Panadol (acetaminophen). After she left, I went to my parents' home. I told my stepfather what happened and he said, "I hope he does not come here and tell us you have been lying." I said, just ask him and our neighbors. At the time I was pregnant, but I was not worried. When my husband came to find me there and my stepfather asked him what happened, he confirmed that he beat me. My parents asked him to divorce me, but he refused.

Women frequently turn upon their families to intervene when their husbands mistreat them. These families, however, must also possess the power and motivation to respond. Few parents would insist on contracts to protect their daughters from their husbands, like her family requested. Many would avoid taking such a public, legal step because it could indicate their inability to mediate their own conflicts. Mairo's stepfather correctly assumed that her husband would hit her again, and this documentation could be used in a court. His reaction reflects the intensity of the violence she experienced.

By withholding her money, Mairo's husband sought to provoke her. Likewise, by refusing to cook her husband's dinner, Mairo demonstrated that she, too, had prepared for a fight. If Nigerians want to offend some-one, they will insult their parents. The flagrancy of this last attack on Mairo prompted the neighbors to intervene. And yet, when the fight was over, one of her neighbors advised her not to leave her husband. Mairo had no intention of staying in his house. Even her stepfather cautioned her not to lie to him. Mairo treaded on territory that few women would venture, as it seemed no one wanted the marriage to end except her.

At the time of this violent encounter, Mairo was full term in her preg-nancy. Soon after, she went to the hospital where her husband worked to deliver the baby. When they got to the maternity ward, her stepfather informed him that Mairo was about to give birth. Her husband said, to her family's shock, that he forbids her from delivering the baby in the hospital. He would not assist her in the costs of medical care. They should take her home. He told them that he would pray for her.

In northern Nigeria, most people believe that husbands have the right to determine whether and where their wives receive medical care because they are responsible for the costs. While, traditionally, it is not unusual for Hausa women to give birth in their homes, Mairo's husband's refusal had nothing to do with Islam or Hausa culture. Instead, Mairo said, his motive was to discipline her for her behavior. As her husband and her stepfather fought in the waiting room, Mairo went into labor. She had not gone for prenatal care and experienced complications as the delivery progressed. She had to have a Caesarian section. In the end, Mairo gave birth to a large, healthy boy. Her husband did not take care of the expenses.

Forty days after she gave birth, Mairo took her husband to a *Shari'a* court.

In court, they asked him if he gave me money for food. He said no. We were told to return after one week. My husband then denied that he had said anything to them. Still, they sent him to jail for a week. On return to the court, I reported that he had never given his son a naming ceremony. The judge ordered him to buy a ram for the naming. He showed up with a skinny one and was told take it back and get another one. He then sent a message to me to send him the head and legs. Of course, I would do no such thing. Back in court, I told the judge what he had said and the judge admonished him. Next, the judge asked me three times if I wanted to return to his house and I said no. He then said to my husband, "I have tried to get [her] to return to your house with no success, so I order you to divorce her." My husband then pronounced a divorce.

Mairo desired an end to her marriage because of her husband's violent temperament and unceasing, brutal discipline. However, courts and families are much more concerned over issues of neglect – particularly over children and subsistence needs. People uniformly agree that these acts are unlawful and inappropriate. Thus, the judge did not focus on instances of physical abuse but rather questions of whether her husband met her needs. Her husband begrudgingly carried out the court's demands. He gave as little to his wife as he possibly could. Still, Mairo had no intention of reconciling. She persisted in her efforts to convince the judge that her husband's behavior was unacceptable. Ultimately, the judge yielded and ordered him to provide her a divorce.

While her mother cautioned her not to say everything she thinks, Mairo would not "swallow" her suffering and remain silent over her husband's egregious abuse. Although her family and the legal system eventually assisted her, they hesitated to end the marriage, preferring the marriage to remain intact regardless of the circumstances. Mairo succeeded in her efforts to escape the marriage. However, her family's ambivalence suggested that she perhaps pushed too hard against the boundaries of her social roles as a wife and a woman. By publicly voicing their problems, she did not exhibit the respectable, dignified behavior expected of wives. Mairo took these lessons to heart in her next marriage.

Mairo's next husband owned a shop close to her family's house in Kano. Prior to her first marriage, this man courted her. "In fact," Mairo said, "we had been in love." After he heard news of the divorce, this boyfriend sent one of his friends to her. He asked, "Was there still something there?" She let him know that she still had feelings for him. Before they could wed, Mairo needed to complete her *iddah*, a three-month waiting period after a woman's divorce. She also had to wean her son. They married five months later. "This time it was a love marriage," Mairo emphasized. Even when married, their former admirers and boyfriends do not disappear from women's lives entirely. Northern Nigerian women all know that marriages rarely last and a woman's marital status does not necessarily deter a man from pursuing her.

Mairo became pregnant with a second child four months after the wedding. Three months after their second son's birth, her husband started to fall sick. He contracted this illness perhaps even prior to their marriage, she said. Her husband hid the symptoms and only took medications at his shop. One day, his friends brought him home. He felt too weak to work. They told her that he lacked the energy to unpack and display his food items. He hired a boy to help him in the shop.

Their relationship then started to sour. Mairo explained,

> My husband's attitude began to change. He started to insult me. Our neighbors were having a ceremony, and my husband came home the night before. He complained that all his clothes were dirty and he had nothing to wear the next day. So I washed the clothes that night. In the morning, he said the sleeves were not clean, so I washed them again and put them on the fan to dry. He continued to complain about how long it would take them to dry. Afterwards, he ironed them while I drew water for his bath. Once dressed, he started insulting me again, stating that my parents, who lived near his business, would not even come to buy things from his shop. He called them paupers. I cried and said, "Well, marriage is not by force. I will go home." When I got there, I told my uncle what happened. He said to wait until his brother comes. Later, we were called for reconciliation. My husband said that my story was not true, but since that is what I said, so be it. I was told to go back inside while he wrote my divorce letter.

Mairo felt deceived, insulted by his comments, and hurt. This man, who she loved very much, behaved similar to her first husband. Based on her experience in that marriage, she did not believe a man's behavior could change despite his promises. Although she was concerned over his sickness, she did not associate these symptoms with HIV. In retrospect, Mairo thought that her husband knew he had already contracted the virus. He sought to end his marriage to keep his status secret. His anger arose from his suspicion that Mairo caused his illness. Because Mairo had no grounds to challenge him, she felt she had to leave.

Two months later, his brother came to plead with Mairo's parents to permit her to return to her husband. Mairo told him that she did not want to return. "His attitude and behavior had shocked me and I no longer wanted to think about him. I told him to tell my husband that I would go find a pauper like me to marry. He should seek an heiress for himself." Her husband persisted in his efforts to make up with Mairo. Because he had only given her a statement of a single divorce, instead of three proclamations, Islam allows reconciliation.

Finally Mairo's mother convinced her to go back to him, "if only for the sake of her child." Upon divorce among Muslims in northern Nigeria, men may claim the right to keep their children after they are weaned. So, Mairo went to his house.

> After some time, he asked me if I knew about AIDS. He then told me his status. I was stunned and exclaimed: "*Inna lillahi wa inna ilaihi raji'un!*" (From God we come and to him we shall return!) I then asked him where he got it. I told him, "You know my first husband does not have it," and he said yes. And then I said, "You know I am not promiscuous either," and again he said that he would vouch for me. He told me that the children and I would be taken to the hospital for tests. The results revealed that the children were negative, but I was positive. From then on, I felt so unhappy. I stopped looking after myself, stopped eating, and turned down invitations to ceremonies. I would tell people that my husband forbids me from attending. They would let me off and blame him instead. I also stopped going to *Islamiyya* (Islamic school) and I even stayed home from graduation. . . . That was when my husband brought me to the doctor. I did not think much about how I got infected. I simply understood that God brought it on us. So, I accepted it. He put the burden on me. That is the fate that was written for me.

When Mairo learned about her husband's diagnosis, she did not consider whether she too had the virus. Instead, she reflexively sought to protect herself from others' accusations. She also became severely depressed. Her fear of being exposed led her to withdraw from her social obligations. Because husbands have the right to forbid their wives from leaving the house, Mairo took advantage of this presumed proscription to justify her absence from these activities. Her husband was complicit in the deceit.

By saying that she chose not to think about their infection, Mairo meant that she would not confront her husband about how he contracted the virus. Instead of accusing him of infecting her, she attributed it to

God's will. Her response contrasted sharply with the protest she raised in her first marriage. Mairo made an implicit bargain: as long as he did not lie and tell others that she infected him with HIV, she would not reveal that he was the one who infected her. In other words, Mairo would keep his betrayal secret.

At this point, Mairo's marital life improved considerably. Just as Jummai's first marriage grew more stable when she assumed responsibility for her husband's secret, so too did Mairo's relationship. She described his affection and care:

> For example, in the mornings we would put *zaitun* (olive oil) and garlic powder in our food. Then we would pray *qul huwal llahu* and *kursiyyu* onto the water we drink. We also ate *habbatu sauda* (black seeds). He would eat so much garlic that, before I cooked, he would send me close to a hundred bulbs to put into the food. It was so much that I used to tease him to find a separate place to keep his clothes because they all smelled of garlic! He replied jokingly, "You mean I should stop coming into the bedroom?"

These loving displays of mutual support continued for almost two more years. Mairo still remained concerned about their health and the well-being of their children. However, her husband – eager to reassert his masculinity by growing his family – persuaded her to have another child.

> He said to me, "Mairo, I am tired of this investment without any returns." And when I became pregnant, he was so happy. . . . The pregnancy was as difficult as my first birth. When I went to the hospital, I was sent for a scan. The doctor advised me to either go for a Caesarian section or take medications to protect the child. Also, I was not supposed to breastfeed when the baby was born. But I simply left everything to God. Another doctor told me I could breastfeed for three months. I knew that at home, my parents would ask why I could not breastfeed. They would assume it was a form of family planning and then my secret might become known. But now, I have weaned him. He is about eighteen months old, though he does not look as strong as the older one. I have been advised to wait until he is two years old before going for an HIV test.

Mairo's desire to conform to the social expectations of motherhood through breastfeeding and a home birth had the additional benefit of masking her illness. This decision, however, put her son's health in danger. She did not have a Caesarian section, nor did she take antiretroviral medications upon the baby's delivery. These measures would have almost certainly improved his chances of receiving an HIV-negative test result. If she had opted not to breastfeed, Mairo thought her family would find out about her status. Alternatively, they might assume that this was a method of family planning, of which they did not approve. Thus, Mairo continued to breastfeed her child, despite her awareness of its possible risks. While their vow to keep each other's secrets may have led to a fleeting feeling of intimacy, the bargain had consequences. It rendered Mairo and her child increasingly vulnerable to poor health.

The tolls that secrets take on women extend beyond threats to their physical well-being. Mairo felt the burden of her secret most acutely soon after she gave birth. Her husband stopped giving her money to care for the children. Seemingly out of nowhere, he began to insult her again. She told me that all of the members of their support group noted this change in his behavior. The doctor who volunteered in the organization that sponsored the group chastised him for his treatment of her. It only grew worse. He would not provide anything for the baby's naming ceremony. He removed his son's bed, clothes, and other items from the house and sold them in his shop. He stopped paying attention to the child whenever Mairo was present.

Furious at Mairo one day, he dismantled her bed and threw her mattress, knitting machine, and other belongings out in the rain. She collected these items and put her bed back in the room. He returned home that evening and asked, "Who brought these things back in the house?" Mairo protested, "You did not even tell me why you took them apart." To that, he said he was tired of the marriage. The terms of their deal had apparently shifted. She did not know what provoked it. She shot back, "Then divorce me because I am no longer the type to run home after quarrels."

I asked Mairo whether she found a new boyfriend after leaving her husband's house. She said:

> In fact, I have already been asked by men for both sex and marriage about four times since then. I tell those who want to marry me that I have not finished my *iddah,* because at the time, I had not. But also, I say it because otherwise everyone will know my secret. I hate my husband for putting me in this position. Our secret would never have to be exposed if we could have remained married and accepted our fate . . . especially with children involved. But he could not.

Mairo lamented her husband's inability to respect their complicit bargain. She feared that her social demise was imminent.

Secrets are enmeshed in power relations between men and women. Mairo illustrated the sacrifices women make as they negotiate these exchanges. By protesting against their husbands' maltreatment, women may encounter the limits of what their networks of families, neighbors, and social institutions – all those charged with the task of protecting them – can provide. Women jeopardize their families' reputations and risk losing everything, including their money, possessions, children, and health, to defend their honor. And yet, by remaining silent, women also uphold a system of masculine privileges that grants men the power to maltreat, abandon, and infect women away from the public's view.

(UN)DIGNIFIED DISCRETION

In northern Nigeria, weddings take place within a larger matrimonial economy, in which symbolic and material exchanges, the formation of new identities, and processes of social reproduction intersect. Nigerians hope to obtain love, dignity, and upward social mobility through marriage. Poor families, in particular, perceive marriage to be an economic, social, and moral refuge for their daughters, especially when they lack the means to support them. However, many men, facing these same economic constraints, cannot or choose not to meet these religious and cultural expectations surrounding marriage. Women's suffering persists as they transition out of their relationships.

Through Jummai and Mairo's narratives, we can identify manifestations of structural violence – that is, the means through which political and economic forces produce deeply entrenched social inequalities. As married women confront the high costs of subsistence, education, and health care while lacking adequate social protections, their dependence on husbands metastasizes. When they do not possess the means, will, or strength to carry out the labor demanded of them within their households, women risk losing everything they value. These inequalities yield violence so embedded in women's everyday lives that their claims for protection from maltreatment are often met with suspicion, blame, and indifference.

Women frequently give more and receive less in their marriages, while these transactions exact painful tolls on their bodies, kin relations, and hopes for the future. As wives seek to protect their well-being, they often strike what I have referred to as patriarchal bargains with their husbands, which appear to further their subordination. In other words, through these unequal exchanges, they implicitly reproduce the same male-centered structures that contributed to their suffering in the first place. Families may be complicit in hiding evidence of the violence that husbands inflict on their wives. With the threat of marital dissolutions persistently lingering, wives must decide how to leverage this secret knowledge for power and protection without jeopardizing already precarious social ties.

In the case of the physical and sexual violence Mairo experienced in her first marriage, she contemplated the following: Do you run away or do you challenge your husband by informing your family and seeking protection from the courts? Or, in the case of her second husband, do you accept that there are things you just cannot know and thus cannot say out loud, much less protest? Is it possible to forge a new kind of intimacy with your husband through sharing a secret? As her second husband ultimately divorced her, Mairo's anger over his betrayal was unambiguous. However, she felt unsure how to proceed in her next relationship.

Likewise, by insisting that she knew all along about her husband's infertility, Jummai attempted to convey that she was neither an ignorant victim nor a "defective" person. As she grew convinced that the disclosure of a shared secret could potentially produce a stable marriage, she attempted – and failed – to secure this trust from her second husband. Her story ended with a pitiable compromise: Jummai once again suffered her husband's illness – and the social scorn that accompanies it – in exchange for a short-lived exchange of money and his acknowledgment that she was not the cause of their infection.

As northern Nigerian women move from marriage to marriage, they must heal from these traumatic betrayals and harmful acts committed by their husbands. They aim to recover their integrity by renewing their efforts to care for their subsequent husbands and families. Strikingly, in Jummai's and Mairo's cases, they see the risk of HIV infection as much less of a threat to their well-being than the lack of a secure footing in their respective marriages. Many HIV-positive women do not know how or from whom they contracted the virus. However, even for those who suspect their current sexual partners have exposed them, they find it difficult, if not impossible, to challenge these men. To do so is to push back against religious and culture norms equating discretion with virtue. And for those currently in relationships, these confrontations may jeopardize the very social resources women are trying to protect. In the next chapter, I consider how the strategic use of speech, silence, and lies becomes a tool through which women aim to enact their respectability.

Dilemmas of Disclosure

Over the past two decades, the number of HIV counseling and testing centers in medical sites across Nigeria has grown exponentially. Women also receive HIV tests when they seek prenatal care in hospitals. Because these services are routinely offered, many wives learn their status without their husbands' knowledge. They must then decide if and how to disclose the results to them. Counselors often complained to me about the difficulties they had trying to persuade women to bring their husbands in for screening. I asked one administrator how she managed this challenge. She told me confidently:

Well, the number one thing that can be done to ease this issue is counseling. When women attend HIV counseling, it goes over very well. But, there is a different way you counsel a man because . . . well, personally, this is the way I do it: I will write a note to the husband. I will say that I would like to see him in the hospital because I have an important issue to discuss with him regarding the baby. So, the moment they see this note, they are very eager . . . that, "a medical personnel wants to see me! Let me go and know what is happening." And, when the man comes, that will be the only opportunity that I have to even sit down and counsel him. . . . Specifically, I tell men, "Okay, when women come to the hospital to deliver the baby, they may need a blood transfusion. And, because HIV is so rampant now, we need to screen your blood." If you just tell men directly that it is an HIV test, they will not like it. You will say that they need to know their blood group, the genotype, and so on. "Without this blood information," we say, "your wife might get blood from somebody, and you will not know whether the person is HIV-positive." They will say, "No! No! No! Madam, please test me so that I will know my status, just in case . . . so that you can prepare for the birth."

I was struck by the fact that this counselor does not tell men directly that she wants them to take an HIV test. She stresses to husbands why the clinic needs to know their blood group and genotype (sickle cell screening) and indirectly references HIV. Then, she solicits their consent through a different tactic: alerting them to the risk of contaminated blood transfusions and persuading them to have their blood screened for donation to ensure their families' safety.

Although national blood policies mandate screening for HIV, hepatitis, and other bloodborne pathogens in health care settings, parents' fear of medical malpractice and neglect is understandable. Nigeria's maternal and infant mortality rates rank among the highest in the world. In effect, the counselor gives men a warning: if you do not receive this test, your children may be infected. By framing the need for screening in this way, the counselor emphasizes a man's responsibility to his wife and children as the rationale for taking a test. Following this cultural logic, she hopes that couples' mutual desire to protect their babies overrides questions of who infected whom.

While this counselor's use of subterfuge may help some people sidestep concerns over who is at fault, women still hesitate to disclose their status to men. Questions about *from whom* and *when* one receives a diagnosis may in fact override concerns surrounding what a test reveals. Women frequently think men will immediately blame them, even if neither of them know the source of the infection. They worry about their security, the possibility of being abandoned, and losing custody of their children. In addition, they think their husbands will disgrace them by revealing their status to the public. Women feel they must wait to disclose until their husbands tell them their own results first. An HIV test, in other words, also reveals their vulnerability.

This chapter evaluates the intersection of speech and power as HIV-positive women navigate the ambiguous terrain of disclosure. What do disclosures *do* – to one's sense of morality, to intimate partnerships, to family relationships, and to life and illness trajectories? While discretion, deception, and exposure may also serve psychological purposes, here I examine the ways in which these disclosures are fundamentally social phenomena: they shape – and are the products of – gender, familial, and deeply moral negotiations.

Acts of speaking do more than just pass along information; saying something out loud has the potential to change social relationships.[1] In the past chapter, Jummai and Mairo's husbands ended their marriages by saying, "I divorce you" aloud to their wives. Most northern Nigerian Muslims recognize this statement of divorce as binding under certain conditions. Speech is also essential to efforts to establish a sense of self. Through performative speech acts, people assume, or are subjected to, an array of characteristics, including their gender, ethnicity, and class, among others.[2] Hausa speakers, for example, use distinctly gendered terms, pronouns, and even styles of laughter to demarcate their identities.[3]

What goes unsaid is just as important as what is said. Victims of violence, for example, may remain silent because they feel their pasts are too shameful or painful to articulate in words. Instead, evidence of trauma is often identified in indirect speech or metaphoric expressions, bodily gestures, and ritual performances. In Nigeria, sufferers often make sense of traumatic experiences through religious idioms, prayer, and other spiritual rites. The women with whom I worked saw discretion as a religious virtue, a means of maintaining stability within their marriage, and a way of protecting their honor. They actively construct and enact silences, rather than passively submitting to them. Likewise, public testimonies may not, in fact, produce solidarity among HIV-positive patients or transcendent experiences of healing and reconciliation. As these women described, disclosures can easily create new rifts in families and communities.[4]

People also use speech to strip others of their sense of self, gender, and morality. In northern Nigeria, I have seen HIV educators misconstrue the actual sources of HIV risk, presenting women as contagious vectors from whom the public must be protected.[5] For example, in 2008, I observed religious and political leaders craft a document titled "National Islamic Policy on HIV/AIDS," in a workshop sponsored by the Nigerian Supreme Council on Islamic Affairs. In it, the leaders referenced two particular prophetic traditions (hadith). First, they write, "The Prophet (SAW) advised a companion to have a proper look at a Madinah woman who(m) he proposed to marry to ascertain that she is free from a defect." And second, in the following section under the heading "Prevention with Positives," they state, "The Prophet (SAW) prohibited people in an epidemic area from leaving the area for fear of infecting others. Caliph Umar directed that the infected should not leave the area nor should uninfected (people) enter the infected area."[6] Although few Nigerians I knew stated these exact hadith, many concurred with these leaders' points.

Similar themes circulate in the popular press. In 2007, the Nigerian newspaper, *This Day,* documented the release of a federally funded report titled *Basic Facts on HIV/AIDS.* The journalist wrote that this report sought to "alert the nation that there were increasing cases of Nigerian ladies who, in their desperate desire to get back at the society . . . dress up provocatively and seek a lift from men, only to end up raping them and gleefully taunt their victims: 'Welcome to the club, you are now HIV-positive.' "[7] In over a decade of work with HIV-infected women, I have not found any evidence to substantiate these claims. Nevertheless, people repeatedly shared these rumors with me. Furthermore, public figures often refer to these maligned representations to justify the exclusion of HIV-positive women from the ordinary pursuits that all women follow, including love and family.

Despite – and sometimes contributing to – these abject portrayals, many authorities attempt to solicit intimate details about HIV-positive women's sexual relationships and livelihoods. These accounts are used for a variety of purposes.[8] Beginning in the late 1990s, public health agencies across Africa sought to foster patient empowerment by introducing a rhetoric of "breaking the silence" within HIV support groups. HIV-positive persons learned to strategically fashion their illness narratives into statements that reflect the values and successes of public health interventions. The heads of these organizations then leveraged patients' testimonials for greater support from donors. Going public, advocates assert, enables HIV-infected persons to join a transnational movement of activists. These global leaders used their presentations to raise awareness and urge support for access to antiretroviral therapies, new medical technologies, and clinical trials. Anthropologists argue that these performances exemplify a form of "therapeutic citizenship." In these public presentations, a patient's personal illness narrative produces political action far more effectively than organizations' claims for resources based on evidence of large-scale processes of structural violence, such as gender inequality or poverty.[9]

Even as HIV-positive diagnoses threatened to discredit their reputations, the women I knew showed little interest in protesting their maltreatment in public. Rather, they directed their energy toward building and affirming kinship ties. Most critically, these efforts included marrying a respectable, supportive man and giving birth to children.[10] If HIV-positive women successfully demonstrate that they can meet these familial expectations, many no longer feel the need to hide their status. Indeed, a number of women stressed to me that they had no difficulty telling others they were HIV positive. They knew they did nothing wrong, as their infection came from their husbands. Consequently, they had nothing to hide. When women cannot meet these kinship ideals, however, they face tremendous challenges. Most women did not openly tell others their status; neither would they reveal the possible social betrayals that resulted in their disease.

Ethics, as I apply the term in this chapter, allows us to link what people say and do to why they think they are doing it. A focus on ethics also permits us to raise questions about the moral and social stakes that women have in these choices and actions. This chapter showcases the ways in which women express and enact ethics through speech. I emphasize how women attempt to effect specific changes in their lives by disclosing some things and withholding others.[11]

LARABA

Laraba, a Muslim divorcee from Kano, had one child from her first marriage before the marriage dissolved. She then entered a polygamous marriage as her new husband's second wife. In 2002, Laraba said she heard on the radio "about a disease that lacked a cure." She worried that her family had contracted the virus. Her husband's first wife, Laraba observed, was never well. She constantly had diarrhea. He also repeatedly fell sick and had rashes all over his body. Soon, Laraba too fell ill.

Anxious to confirm her suspicion, Laraba told her husband that she wanted to go to the hospital. Although she did not tell him that she wanted

an HIV test, he refused to take her there or provide money for transportation. Without his knowledge, she asked her parents for help. By emphasizing her husband's lack of support, I think Laraba was pointing two things
out to me: first, he violated the Islamic expectation that men take care of
their wives' health and, second, she knew that he would deny his illness
if she received a positive test result. Laraba said she anticipated a major
conflict in their household, implying that her husband already might have
known the cause of their illness.

At the hospital, the physician ordered tests for malaria and typhoid,
two of the most common illnesses in northern Nigeria. The pharmacist
gave her malaria medications; however, she did not improve. She returned
to the hospital, and they conducted another test. This time, they did not
explicitly tell Laraba the purpose of their screening. In 2002, pretest counseling for HIV was not mandatory, as it is today. Physicians screened many
women for the virus without their knowledge. Laraba said:

> When I went back a week later to collect the result, I overheard the doctor
> telling the interpreter that some woman was HIV-positive. When I reached
> her table, I saw that the card in front of her had my name on it. She then
> asked me if I understood English. I said no. She would not say what was
> wrong and told me to go back to the lab. At the lab, the technician got me
> a chair and asked if I wanted some water. He made sure we would not be
> disturbed. He then asked me my name and if I had a husband. I told him
> yes – and a son, also. He began to preach and said I should understand that,
> "All that happens to humans is as God wishes." He asked me if I had
> heard about the "incurable disease" on the radio and I said yes. So, he said,
> "That is what you have." He said to tell my husband that he was needed
> at the hospital, but not to tell him my status or the reason why he was
> needed. . . . Honestly, I did not feel much then. The doctor said that there
> were no HIV medications. I should just continue to come to the clinic.

Laraba began her narrative by emphasizing how she feigned an inability
to understand English. This decision could be interpreted in a number
of ways. It is possible that she lacked the confidence to discuss such an
important medical concern in English. She preferred to learn the result
of her test in Hausa. Many people feel intimidated in hospitals. I observed
patients frequently remain silent in their consultations with physicians,
nurses, and even counselors, asking few, if any, questions. Although north-

ern Nigerians primarily speak Hausa, I found that men and women often understood more English than they allowed me to know. Likewise, I also occasionally let people assume I understood less Hausa than I actually knew because I wanted to hear what people said about me behind my back. Silences may allow us to gain access to knowledge and, consequently, power, not otherwise given away freely.

However, I suspect that Laraba concealed her comprehension of English not simply to elicit a greater understanding of her illness. This is also a particularly useful tactic to uncover information physicians and nurses might withhold from her. Furthermore, this disguise might have allowed her to distance herself from the responsibilities associated with this knowledge. In other words, Laraba likely sought to establish a position of plausible deniability. By claiming ignorance about the disease and her diagnosis, she avoids accusations of failing to take accountability for the family's health.

In northern Nigeria, women are disproportionately vulnerable to such accusations. Laraba may also not have trusted the medical staff. Would they tell her if she was dying? What else would they hide from her? Would they disclose her illness to others without her knowledge? Would they inform her husband? Of course, when patients raise these questions, counselors quickly try to curb their anxieties. They assure them that their private information will remain confidential. Hospital policies prohibit them from sharing files without permission. Even without these assurances, Laraba's access to this information likely provided her a sense of control over an otherwise precarious situation.

In addition to Laraba's concealed knowledge, I was surprised by the technician's reluctance to call her disease HIV. I later learned that this oblique manner of speaking was quite common. Hausa speakers often use indirect speech to refer to an array of issues, especially terms related to the body, sexuality, and disease. Laraba and the technician undoubtedly knew the meaning of "that disease without a cure." As he set the scene for his disclosure, the technician did not address the behaviors that exposed her to the virus. Instead, he sought to mitigate Laraba's anxiety and console her.

Because this theme echoed across many HIV-positive women's narratives, I pressed another of my informants to help me understand it better.

She said, "All diseases are destiny. God gave you the disease in order to forgive you. God says He never gives you one trouble without taking away another from you; that is, if God gave people this disease, there is another thing he will relieve them of." By drawing on this Islamic tenet, the laboratory technician aimed to normalize HIV as one of any number of threats to Laraba's health and well-being. He presented a moral interpretation to her: the disease may, in fact, produce something good in her future. Laraba should therefore not worry about how or why she contracted the virus. Put another way, an HIV test could reveal God's plans for a person's life.

I do not think Laraba had any doubt that her husband infected her. Nevertheless, she and the technician implicitly knew that her positive diagnosis posed a significant risk to her personal safety and her marriage if her husband learned her status. He already behaved suspiciously by forbidding Laraba from going to the hospital. Either he did not prioritize her health or he knew more about this illness than he would share with her. By defying him, Laraba revealed her readiness to face the consequences of this breach and her assuredness that she could follow through with the test without his knowledge. However, disclosure presented a much greater danger.

The technician colluded with Laraba in an act of subterfuge. They lured her husband to the laboratory with a tactic similar to the one used by the counselor in the introduction. When she arrived at home that day, Laraba nonchalantly said to her husband that the physician asked him to come to the hospital. He agreed but then delayed. Later, when Laraba reminded him about the request, her husband angrily questioned whether the physician told her that he caused her sickness. She said they told her nothing.

When Laraba and her husband finally went to the hospital together, she informed the staff discreetly that he did not know about her HIV test. The physician then lied to her husband and said to him that he was concerned about Laraba's difficulty in conceiving a baby. They wanted to run some tests on him as well to diagnose the problem. After the test, one of the hospital's staff members led them to the lab technician's office. Laraba's husband wanted her to leave, but the technician said that they should both stay. He counseled them in English: "He told us there is no cure. He advised us to eat well and we would be able to live with the virus longer." Laraba continued:

> When we left the office, I asked my husband what was wrong. I told him
> that I pretended to understand what the man said, but in reality, I did not.
> This, I did just to test him. He said the illness was not a problem. There is a
> woman who was taken to an herbalist and was cured, so he would go get us
> medications from him. So, my husband concluded, "Our illness is nothing
> to worry about."

As I listened to Laraba's story, I suspected that her husband hesitated to go to the hospital because he knew his status all along. Just as the counselor suggested, a man's concern over his wife's reproductive health might motivate him to agree to an HIV test when he otherwise would evade it. His reluctance to have his wife present when they notified him of his results suggested to me that he did not want her to know what, if anything, was wrong. Perhaps sensing his wariness, Laraba continued with the pretense of not understanding enough English to follow the discussion. Her husband took advantage of this feigned ignorance and lied to her about their diagnosis. He simply said he would take care of it.

Laraba then stressed to me that her husband told her there was a cure, which we both knew was wrong. By emphasizing this point, I think Laraba attempted to frame his behavior to me in moral terms: what kind of husband would lie to his wife in such an egregious way? He was not merely avoiding calling HIV by its name; he was denying outright that HIV was the source of their illness.

I asked Laraba what happened after that. She said,

> Without him knowing, I told my parents what happened. My dad heard
> about a traditional medicine and he bought it for me. By God's grace, I
> started getting better. I regained my strength, even though I knew the
> disease was still there. I then offered it my husband. He was suspicious,
> but I told him that it was from my father. He began taking it. After a
> while, I told him that the herbalist said my co-wife should also take the
> medicine. But, my husband then said she was okay. I asked him, "What do
> you mean that this woman is okay?" He said, "You know it is just fever."
> So I said, "Fine." After finishing the medicine, my father asked me if all
> three of us were taking it. I told him no. He said, "Talk to your husband
> because, if she dies, then you are at fault. You have cheated her." I spoke

to my husband again and he asked why I bothered him about the issue. I should just stay away from her.

Laraba continued to hide her knowledge and actions from her husband and instead told her parents, who immediately came to her assistance. For some HIV-positive women, parents play formidable roles in mediating their daughters' disclosures. Their efforts to find Laraba an effective treatment showed not just their concern for her health but also, I believe, her marriage. If Laraba's illness worsened, her neighbors, friends, and other family members would know that her husband was not caring for her. In other words, without medications, symptoms would not simply appear on her body; her poor health would reveal her husband's maltreatment. Laraba's parents also provided her medicines to give to her husband and co-wife. This, however, put her in a difficult ethical position.

Laraba knew that if she gave her husband and co-wife this treatment, she would give away her secret. The action would reveal that she knew her status and that she hid this knowledge from her husband. Yet, if she did not intervene, she would watch them both grow ill, while she possessed a treatment that could palliate their suffering. Laraba responded by showing her husband that she was invested in caring for him, while denying she knew anything about the medication itself. However, in northern Nigeria, co-wives' relationships are often characterized by jealousy, suspicion, and ambivalence, at best. Laraba would thus have a far more difficult time convincing her mate to take a traditional medicine for an unnamed illness.

Parents often intervene in conflicts between their daughters and co-wives, but Laraba's father took an unusually firm stance. He rejected the cultural expectation that co-wives should mind their own business, impressing on Laraba that she is obligated to take care of them. It sounded to me like her father uttered this statement in the form of a threat: if she does nothing, she will face the consequences of her inaction in the future. Laraba's father knew she had not disclosed her status to her husband and co-wife. He did not approve. This threat served as a reminder that he also possessed power, which she must respect. Laraba delayed as long as she could, waiting to see if her husband would change his stance and confide in them. As he showed no sign of yielding, she ultimately conceded.

Laraba approached her co-wife and gave her the medications. She did not, however, tell her that HIV made her sick. Laraba concluded:

> I gave her the medicine, but she was upset that our husband would be so hypocritical. I do not know whether she quarreled with him or what, but the next day he stopped talking to me completely. This went on for three months. I just kept to myself. Whenever I asked him why he is not speaking with me, he would deny that he was angry. Next, he stopped giving me money to visit the clinic, and both he and his wife stopped taking the medication. Her illness became so bad that she could not get out of bed. When he returned from work, he would go and chat with her. That was it. I finally lost my patience and I told him I was tired of this business. He should just divorce me. My husband said, "Since you have said so, I will tell you your offense toward me: You are not trustworthy." Then he said, "I am also tired of being married to you," and he divorced me.

Laraba grappled with a number of competing concerns over whether and how to disclose her knowledge to her co-wife. First, she unquestionably feared her father's condemnation. She would breach a moral code if she withheld these medications and watched her family members suffer. And yet, she also knew that women should not intervene in affairs between their co-wives and husbands. More important, Laraba sensed the marriage would end if she exposed her husband's secret.

Laraba attempted to avoid these risks by giving the other wife medications without naming the illness. This was such an extraordinary gesture, however, that her co-wife immediately suspected her motives. Laraba had no opportunity to reconcile with her, as she and her husband ignored Laraba from that point onward. Met with her husband's silence and cut off from his support, she chose not to do or say anything more about their diagnosis.

Anticipating that their deaths were near, Laraba felt her only recourse was to ask her husband for a divorce. Unsurprisingly, he accused her of being untrustworthy. Because she could not keep their illness secret, he ended the marriage. Laraba's husband never disclosed his status to her, nor did she disclose hers to him.

MERCY

In the city of Jos over spring 2003, I met with Mercy, a lab technician. She was a widow with two young daughters and the first HIV-positive person I had ever interviewed in Nigeria. In the early years of their relationship, Mercy and her husband worked diligently for respectable and lucrative occupations. She said he dreamed that the Lord directed him to the Uni-Petrol oil company in Lagos. He applied and they offered him a job. Not long after, Mercy gave birth to a baby girl. When her husband's company transferred him to Kano, Mercy returned to Jos to care for the child.

Over a year passed, and he did not return. Mercy was surprised by his change in behavior. When he finally came back for a short visit, he spent the night out with his friends. Mercy asked, at one point, if she could visit him in Kano, and this request was met with rebuke and a violent ultimatum: she should never come to see him there. Mercy backed off.

Just as in Laraba's case, it is clear that conflicts between husbands and wives are performative; people use language to convey multiple meanings and intentions, as well as transform social roles and situations. These efforts may be explicit. For example, Mercy *did* in fact want to move to Kano. However, these statements contain unspoken meanings, as well. Mercy intended to let her husband know she desired reconciliation. At the same time, she conveyed her suspicion over his behavior.

Likewise, Mercy's husband's threat did more than inform her she was unwelcome in Kano. Although he did not say what would happen to her, he implied that he would take action. This hostile statement served to remind Mercy of his dominance. Furthermore, it intimated his willingness to harm her if she defied him. Speech acts, in other words, may dispossess people of power and virtue, just as they can produce these same resources.

As Mercy's marriage unraveled, her in-laws and community learned about her husband's infidelity. She heard rumors that he lived with another woman. His family attributed his affair to the fact that Mercy had not given birth to a son. Her mother-in-law defended her son and insulted her. She told Mercy that she was a "nothing." His family encouraged her husband to end his marriage with her and marry another woman. They downplayed his transgressions through unconcealed accusations against her.

Mercy's in-laws further consolidated their social ties by excluding her from their family through the use of gossip. Specifically, they reworked evidence of her husband's abuse into a narrative about Mercy's inability to uphold the moral norms expected of her as a wife. These insinuations also served as a diversion. They allowed her husband to hide these relationships while simultaneously silencing Mercy. Her protests would only reaffirm her reputation as a wayward wife. And finally, these exchanges foreshadowed his family's ability to fabricate stories about the cause of her husband's illness and the maltreatment Mercy would face after his death.

Despite their strained relationship, her husband occasionally returned to Jos, and they resumed having sex. Much to her relief, Mercy became pregnant. She thought that her husband would finally pay attention to her. He then flatly denied that the baby belonged to him. In effect, her husband accused her of infidelity. Just as northern Nigerian Muslims establish a divorce through a spoken act, Mercy husband's rejection of his parentage was an indirect attempt to dissolve the relationship through speech.

Up until now, Mercy remained resolute in her discretion, hiding her anger and humiliation. This time, she argued back, "It cannot work! I married you when you had nothing. Now you are 'something' and you want me to leave. Where do you want me to go? I cannot go back to my parents' house. I will stay even if you want to remarry. I will stay." Mercy refused to be abandoned. She decided to follow her husband to Lagos, where he had recently been transferred.

Mercy's husband relented and begrudgingly found her a room in the city. He moved into another apartment, presumably with one of his girlfriends, she speculated. In response to her antagonistic attitude, her husband flaunted his money and his affairs. He refused to give Mercy anything. She had no money to attend a prenatal clinic. Unknown to her, he learned that he had contracted the virus at this time. Whether intentional or not, his outward antipathetic behavior probably masked his anxiety and suffering, Mercy suggested. Eventually, her husband's body began to betray his secret. He had lost his job, and his health was rapidly deteriorating.

In October 2000, she brought him to a hospital, and the doctors admitted him. Mercy described to me how she obtained his HIV test results:

> I went and met the doctor and asked him, "What is the problem with my husband?" He said that there was nothing wrong. He will soon be OK. "Just tell me," I insisted, "I am a medical personnel. No matter how serious the case is. . . ." He asked, "You are a medical personnel?" I told him, "Yes, we work on these kinds of cases. That is why I came to ask." I told him that I am going to leave my husband with him. If anything happened to him, he should contact his family and tell them – because I do not want to try to answer questions when I do not know anything about his situation. . . . "If he dies, do not ever look for me because I will sue you." The doctor was scared. He said, "Madam, I am sorry but your husband is HIV positive. Do not tell him I told you. He warned me that I should never tell you; he did not know how you would take it."

Mercy framed her need to know his status in the form of a direct threat to the doctor: if her husband dies, her in-laws will ask her for information, and she refuses to be an intermediary in this exchange. The doctor should be afraid of the family's response, Mercy implied, not just because his patient fell sick and died without the family's knowledge but also because the hospital deliberately hid the diagnosis. If the doctor solicited her help in counseling them, Mercy claimed that she would sue him. Swayed, perhaps, both by Mercy's efforts to show she is his equal – that she deals with cases like this in her work – and the possibility of the family taking action against him, the doctor finally disclosed her husband's status.

As we spoke that day, I felt certain that Mercy suspected her husband was HIV-positive all along. Why not ask him directly? Why go through so much trouble to secure this information from the doctor? She never mentioned to me that she was concerned about her own status or even whether HIV caused her daughter's illnesses at that point. Most critical to Mercy was that she got his diagnosis before her in-laws could. She knew they would blame her, just as they had for his infidelity. If she found out his test results before her husband became aware of it, she could use this information to protect herself from his family's accusations.

Although her husband finally turned to Mercy for care, she had no reason to believe he would protect her. After learning his diagnosis, Mercy wasted no time letting his family know why he was sick. Alarmed by this news and afraid she would expose his status to their community, his family relented in their abuse. Because she did not appear sick, and because she had not been tested, Mercy could deny she was the source of his illness.

Her husband's family decided they would lie and say someone poisoned him. This time, Mercy was not left out of the secret. By colluding with his in-laws in their fabricated story, she acquired greater power. His positive status threatened to shame the entire family, and she was the only person who possessed irrefutable evidence of the diagnosis. Her complicity provided her a means of relating to his in-laws in a new way, where she was respected as a person equally invested in the care of their son.

By taking on this arduous responsibility, I suspect that Mercy also wanted to prove that she was capable of upholding the moral norms expected of all Nigerian wives in their households. If she could accomplish this, she might finally attain her dignity. Mercy left her job as a laboratory technician to provide him full-time attention. She administered intravenous medications and cleaned up his vomit and defecation. He could not walk.

Although his sisters also came to help, Mercy did not want them to go near his fluids. "I did not want them to get involved because they are still very young. I did not want their future to be ruined," Mercy said, referring to her fear that they would contract the virus. At this point, she likely knew that she too had HIV, but she could not – or would not – say it out loud.

A week before he died, Mercy's husband called her over to him. He wanted to apologize, he said. He confessed that he had hurt her and he wanted her forgiveness. Although she knew that he was referring to HIV, Mercy confronted him, "What are the things you did to me?" He said that he had known he was infected for over two years. The company provided money for his medical care, but instead, he gave it to his younger brother to pay for his wedding. He disclosed not only his HIV status but also the other secrets he and his family had attempted to hide. These included his extramarital relationships, alcoholism, and his profligate spending habits. "He did not want to tell me because he knew I would be hurt," Mercy said. "There was nothing I could do then, but to forgive him."

Disclosures do not just passively convey information. They may be couched in the form of apologies and laden with regret, guilt, and fear. Mercy demanded explicit acknowledgment that she was a virtuous wife. Her husband believed, perhaps disingenuously, that women are incapable of hearing such devastating news. He thought his deception protected her. His confession provided Mercy vital information about her health and the well-being of her family. She also felt that it validated her moral claims. In turn, her husband's statement gave Mercy the power to forgive him. This act of forgiveness may have been offered in exchange for the "gift" of a fleeting experience of intimacy.

Mercy tearfully narrated his last days. She explained to me that she had never experienced a death in her family before:

> On Friday, around 7 p.m., my husband called me to ask his half-brother to go see him. Once we were together, he said we should bring our hands. I held hands with him and his brother. He said, "These kids that you have . . . please take good care of them for me." I just looked at him. He told his brother, "David, take care of my wife." My friends were there. I just laughed and said, "Look at the way he is talking!" I did not know he was saying goodbye. After that, he could not talk. . . . Early in the morning, around 1:50, I heard him struggling to breathe. I was sleeping, but not deep. Before I got to him, he was dead.

The exchanges unfolding over the days and hours before Mercy's husband's death illustrate how language, intimacy, and power intersect. These conversations contrasted sharply with the indirect disclosures that Mercy elicited from her husband over the course of their relationship. Their initial "game" of reputation management was fraught with an inordinate amount of suffering, duplicity, and bad faith. Through this final display of their mutual desire to care for one another, Mercy and her husband briefly stood on equal footing. While she may have experienced the moment as a gift of an apology in exchange for her forgiveness, this disclosure, nevertheless, only happened at a point when her husband's impending death stripped him of his power. He had nothing left to lose.

After Mercy's husband passed away, she fell back into disputes with her in-laws over her inheritance and her daughters' custody. Her husband's family told everyone that Mercy poisoned him. They blamed her for his death and forbade her from leaving town with her children. Frustrated and disgusted, Mercy rejected their character assaults by remaining silent: "Because of my problem [HIV], I did not want to add more stress. I just kept quiet." However, the community's hostility, coupled with the loss of her husband and her job, took its toll. Mercy felt utterly stripped of her dignity. Finally, she sought a test. The counselor confirmed that she and her youngest daughter were HIV-positive. Mercy said, from that moment, she no longer hid the fact that she was HIV-positive. The disease was her fate.

While both Mercy and her husband experienced a loss of face after their diagnosis, there are crucial differences in their disclosures to others. Her husband's disclosure allowed him to accomplish a number of things. For one, he belatedly reassured Mercy that she was, in fact, an honorable wife. This acknowledgment symbolically communicated his gratitude. In addition, her husband's plea for his children's care demonstrated his concern for his family – a gesture that inspired Mercy's forgiveness. For Christians and Muslims alike, forgiveness serves an important spiritual function, particularly when one is near death. Thus, her husband endeavored to display his integrity in this final act.

Mercy, conversely, gained little when she first received her test results. Her friends no longer visited after they learned her status. Members of her church avoided her. Her in-laws and pastor absconded with her share of her husband's death benefits from his employer, as well as their children's inheritance. Mercy also blamed herself for the death of her mother, who she claimed was overwhelmed by the stress of her diagnosis. Nonetheless, with the assistance of physicians and hospital donors, Mercy located HIV medications for herself and her daughter. Although she was not aware of it at the time of her diagnosis, she would eventually be able to leverage these health care resources into a new set of social relations as the founder of an HIV support group in 2002.

HALIMA

In 2010, I sat with a shy Muslim woman named Halima in a quiet office of the treatment center where she collected her medication each month. Halima was from Kano and had been married twice before with two children, who lived with her parents in Kaduna. She insisted on conducting the interview in English, even though Hausa was her first language. The focus of this particular session was on women's beauty routines and their bodies. As we proceeded, however, our discussion veered in a different direction.

Noting that Halima looked not only healthy but also very pretty, I asked, "If a man sees a beautiful girl, what does he like?" She did not offer me a long list of physical features or personality traits, as many women did. Halima also did not describe her own characteristics, which men undoubtedly admired, I thought. Instead, she echoed my reference to the categories of "men" and "girls" and told me a vivid story about a couple, using the pronouns *he* and *she*. It was not clear to me whether this couple was a specific pair of individuals whom she knew or an abstract exemplar she created to address my question. She began, "First, a man sees a girl he likes. He says, 'Hi baby.' He says, 'Fine baby. Come. Let me help you reach where you are going.' He has a car. If the girl agrees, she follows him to his car. He tells her he wants to take her to a restaurant. Before long, he has bought things like yogurt, chicken, eggs, and so on."

I asked, "The man spends money on the lady?"

"He buys a lot of things for the girl. The girl has already melted inside. Anything he says, she will agree. He will tell her, 'Let me take you to my house.' She will follow him."

Halima trailed off. "What happens after that?" I prompted.

"He will tell her to lie on his bed. She will not object. He will kiss her, romance her, anything. Then he will make love to her. Anything could happen to the girl. She does not know his HIV status."

As we continued, Halima elaborated on how the man infects his girlfriend without her knowledge. He deceives her by showering her family with gifts. Because this man is not married, she said, he routinely visits his many girlfriends. He avoids meeting her family in person and attempts to keep his girlfriends from knowing about each other. "He likes beautiful girls," Halima pointed out. "He has a weakness for them."

Religious and popular discourses across the country present premarital and extramarital sexual relationships as both immoral and dangerous. However, many men take great pride in their ability to provide for both their wives and girlfriends. Like Halima stated, attractive boyfriends may own cars and offer their girlfriends expensive gifts. Even if they lack a stable salary or savings, men may attempt to fool their girlfriends into believing they are rich.

Men's notion of respectability is further buttressed by their control over women's sexuality. In Halima's terms: "The girl has already melted inside.

Anything he says, she will agree." Men employ these elaborate displays of affluence to seduce girlfriends into having sex with them. These sexual relationships are public secrets – that is, social facts that are widely known but never spoken about.[12] Many women rationalize these relationships as an effect of men's inability to resist their sexual impulses.

Following her thoughts about men's weakness for women, Halima explained that this woman, in fact, cares only for the man's money. Because her parents are poor, she gives her family his gifts – food, money, and other items. These generous gestures make them reluctant to question whether this boyfriend is serious about his marriage intentions. Halima explained that if the parents begin to suspect otherwise, they will be angry and take her to the hospital for an HIV test. "If she has HIV, the parents are as good as dead." In other words, her parents will disown her. She will then leave the house, "looking for and following men."

Halima continued:

If the HIV-positive girl is dirty [or her appearance is unkempt] and not feeling fine, a boy might approach her. He will start to wonder if this is the Aisha, or Zainab or Hajara, whom he knew when he was younger. . . . She says it is she! He asks her what is wrong with her and what she is doing. He offers to take her to his house. She follows him, takes her bath, and eats. He gives her everything she needs . . . she will then tell him lies. She will say her parents are dead and she has no one. But this woman will know her HIV status and he will not know his. She will continue to sleep with him. After some time, she will start looking good again because she is taking proper care of herself. She will go and see other men and spread the virus, all the while she knows her status.

When a woman finds a man she wishes to marry, Halima explained, she hides her status from him. The husband eventually finds out once she becomes pregnant: "The husband will become so happy that his wife is going to have a baby. Then, the hospital will want to test the wife because of the baby. The husband collects the form and looks at what happened. *She lives dangerously.* She was sleeping with all kinds of men before he came to marry her. She knows her status."

I probed Halima for more details about the woman: did she disclose to him that she had HIV? Halima surmised: no. She will not ever tell him and he will eventually widow her.

As Halima proceeded, however, she complicated the moral judgments cast upon HIV-positive women and their sexual lives. She changed topics from women's sexual transgressions to the effects of men's adultery on the well-being of their wives and children. Next, she emphasized men's power in their choice of sexual partners. Because the woman needs money to care for her HIV-infected baby, Halima explained, "Maybe she keeps following men to survive and these men too have their own wives. Some two, some four, and she too has other men on the side. She infects the men and the men infect their many wives at home."

When the woman's new boyfriend falls ill, he returns home and the burden of care falls upon his wives: "Today, he is sick. Tomorrow, he is a bit better. He messes himself and his old wives clean him up and change his clothes. If he does not go to the hospital, he dies at home and leaves behind his wives, family, in-laws, and so on."

Halima's gaze seemed to wander. She spoke quietly, "So before you pick girls, always think of the family you have at home. He should think well." Halima then repeated to me that the man's entire family contracted HIV as a result of his extramarital affairs.

Halima initially suggested that men could not resist their attraction to beautiful women. Yet, when she cautions the man in her narrative to "think well" before he pursues girlfriends, Halima indicates men do, in fact, possess agency. As she gained confidence in this point, Halima articulated how the moral imperative of responsible motherhood, wifehood, and self-care trumps taboos over HIV-positive women's sexual relationships:

> You test your newborn baby. If it is negative, the doctor can give you ideas on how to keep your child from getting sick. If you have the sickness, eat well, do not think too much, do not do overly hard work, keep yourself neat . . . all will be fine. If you do not have the money, why will you not work to feed yourself? If not, anything can happen tomorrow. Some people in Nigeria have no house, yet they have plenty of children. They give birth every year. They have no food to eat and no money for school. If you are sick, what do you do?

Here, Halima aims to cement her own ethical subjectivity to me as one woman among many in Nigeria and around the world – concerned about their families' health and economic well-being. Her narrative accomplishes two things: first, by repeating her earlier description of wives' struggles, she highlights how nonmarried HIV-positive women, including married men's lovers, also dutifully care for themselves, their partners, and their families. This point, once again, reflects her emphasis on the virtues all women seek to display, regardless of their marital or HIV status.

Second, Halima shifts from a vague use of *she* and *he* to the impersonal use of the pronoun *you*. Uttered in the tone of a timid caution, she ostensibly directs her first use of "you" toward married men, warning them to be mindful of their families before they pursue girlfriends. Halima then assumes a more assertive voice as she appears to address an audience that could refer to her society, more broadly.

Like the pronoun *one* in English or other impersonal pronouns such as /on/ in French or /a/ in Hausa, a speaker uses an impersonal *you* to state a generally accepted truth or an opinion that she believes others share. Speakers also switch to this voice to identify categories of persons to which they belong. In other words, as people employ impersonal pronouns to describe what typically occurs in a given situation – an event that could occur to anyone – it often means they also have shared this experience.[13] By speaking without specifics, I think that Halima aimed to transform a story rife with parallels to popular discourses about the perilous sexual lives of HIV-positive women to that of "everyman" and "everywoman."

Halima's use of "you" also links the particular problem of HIV-infected women's sexual decisions to the larger social problem of poverty. Rather than passively accepting these economic circumstances, she questions, how could any woman not do everything she can to earn money for her children? While men gain greater social status for fully providing for their children, Halima responds that women too attain virtue through work. This labor is an extension of their maternal responsibilities. The shift in grammatical person from the generic *he/she* to the impersonal *you* suggests to me that there is more to Halima's story than its literal meaning. She challenges these invidious narratives about HIV-positive women by offering a different framing.

After raising the question, "What do you do?" Halima paused and waited for a response from me. I said nothing. She continued,

> This is the problem. After my husband died, I left his house. For almost five years, I did all kinds of work: cleaning, selling water . . . anything to

buy my children food. I sold bean cakes. I sold food in motor parks and on the roadside. I did everything just to get money to feed us.

Then I replied, "But it's not enough?" "It's not enough," Halima said. She explained, "Before my husband died . . . all our money was spent trying to care for him. He was not strong enough to work. We used our money to buy food and drugs. The money finished (was used up) even before he died. *After he died, I went to a very dangerous life.*"

Halima's grammatical voice had shifted to the first person and she spoke in the past tense. This discursive move finally established herself as a participant in the story. However ambiguous her language, I believe she was an actor in the narratives she presented to me from the very beginning of our interview.

Halima contracted the virus but felt fine. She worked hard to eat well and not worry. She kept herself neat. Halima had children and struggled to earn money to feed them. As a widow, she had no other option but to pursue jobs many northern Nigerians consider disreputable. Halima sold food at public transportation hubs, mainly occupied by male drivers and passengers. These sites also attract other sordid characters involved in illicit or questionable activities. In addition, this work rarely provides women a sufficient income. By repeating the phrase "a dangerous life," Halima indirectly identified herself as one of many HIV-positive women who have sex in exchange for economic support.

As we continued, Halima elaborated on the hardships she encountered after her first husband's death. She could not rely on her parents, and her close friends lacked employment. She worried about paying her children's school fees. Halima occasionally withdrew them from school because she had no money. I asked her how she met her current husband and the support he provided.

> He told me he already had a wife, but he wants to marry me. I said, "No problem. I like you, too." I told him I had children. He said he did not mind. I told him I had nothing and I was responsible for my children. He said, "No problem. When we marry, you can care for your kids." After I married him, he said I am not allowed to bring my children into his house. I should stay at home and not go anywhere. Then, I brought the children to my mother in Kaduna. At home, I sell earrings, bangles, and other jewelry, eyeliner, and so on. If I sell things, I have money to care for my children.

My husband does not know that I sell these things. If he knew, he would be angry.

Halima explained to me that she did not get along with her co-wife. She felt her husband treated her unfairly. He refused to give her money because he suspected she would spend it on her children in Kaduna instead of the household. He spent all of his money on his first wife and her children, she said.

Halima was then four months pregnant with his child. She feared he would not even give her money to purchase formula. During her last pregnancy with her former husband, she sold her clothes to buy milk for their baby. At the time of our interview, she was considering terminating the pregnancy. Halima told me that her second husband is currently infected, along with her co-wife. She did not say whether she knew she was infected prior to their engagement.

As a woman and a person infected with HIV, Halima occupies a doubly marginalized position in northern Nigerian society. Even as she sought to protest the circumstances that expose women to HIV and deny them the means to adequately protect children, she still confronted the limits of what she could say aloud. And, indeed, like many women who experience violence, neglect, and abuse in their relationships, Halima felt deeply and understandably reluctant to narrate these experiences.

Halima circumnavigated the potential repercussions of identifying herself as one of these women, through her prose. In switching from the third-, to second-, to first-person voice over the course of our conversation, Halima addressed entrenched and largely taken-for-granted moral discourses about deceitful and undignified women who the public blames for the spread of HIV in Nigeria. In their place, she offers a narrative in which she presents herself as a virtuous subject, who acts as any woman would act. Put differently: *These circumstances can happen to anyone. It can happen to you. It happened to me.*

As anthropologists collect personal narratives, our research subjects simultaneously assess our knowledge, experience, and the stances we take on particular concerns.[14] In the beginning, Halima presented a narrative that I would undoubtedly recognize given how widespread these public discourses circulate. I believe she watched me to see whether I would agree with the popular and religious sentiments she referenced. This knowledge would afford her the option to withdraw from the interview entirely if she sensed a threat. Halima negotiated this uncertainty through the strategic use of speech.

By moving from a third-person experience to a firsthand account, Halima lends credibility to her argument. She could not or chose not to detail the difficult sexual decisions she made to secure support for herself and her children. Instead, she establishes and prolongs the ambiguity between her past behavior and her present situation.

Yet, her narrative clearly reveals what is at stake in these transactions. Through her spoken and unspoken testimony, Halima expresses her anger, sense of violation, and feelings of powerlessness. At the same time, she offers a profound illustration of women's agency in the context of formidable structural constraints. Her ability to "tell but not tell" hints at her personal struggles but also at how speech itself becomes a form of social and ethical engagement.

GRAMMATICAL PERSONHOOD

HIV disclosures, as I have described, are speech acts. They do far more than simply present information to listeners. HIV-positive women uniformly contend that the timing of disclosure is crucial. Context matters. Women further insist that it is important they learn their husbands' results first. When a husband and wife finally exchange this information, some couples experience greater intimacy and even a sense of equality within the marriage. In addition, they may communicate their gratitude and personal integrity, thus inspiring forgiveness. Nevertheless, too often people disclose their status when they have nothing left to lose. If disclosures go awry, women are far more likely than men to jeopardize the little capital they possess. Thus, many women say nothing.

Silences, like disclosures, are performative. They unfold in the context of other speech acts. For example, in Hausa, people not only speak obliquely about HIV – "the disease without a name" – but also about bodies, sex, and illness, among others. In this chapter, Halima offered an open-ended story of a couple whose identity was unknown to me but

whose actions sounded analogous to popular tropes about the dangerous sexuality of HIV-positive women. Using a third-person voice, she
distanced herself from the description she provided, yet still guided
me to a conclusion that these tropes do not typically reach.

Silences also reflect and shape the power an individual possesses.
On one hand, they allow us to gain access to knowledge otherwise un-
available. HIV-positive women, like Laraba, strategically employ silence
to establish plausible deniability. If they do not know their status, no one
will accuse them of failing to respond in ways they cannot. On the other
hand, husbands and their families may conspire to silence women to deny
them the opportunity to defend themselves against their abuses. Silence
is therefore not merely the absence of speech. However potent the substance of a woman's knowledge, it may not offer sufficient protection when
other structural inequalities strip her of the ability to raise her voice.

To forestall the consequences of saying too much or saying too little,
HIV-positive women lie. Lies express much more than untrue statements.
They are socially shared and performed and serve a variety of purposes. For
example, counselors and their clients engage in subterfuge to convince
men to take a blood test. They achieve this by replacing a clinical rationale
for testing with a cultural rationale. HIV-infected wives can then circumvent power structures that prevent them from confronting their husbands
directly. As accomplices in these lies, women are tied with people who
share this knowledge. Access to damaging information may also provide
women protection from retaliation.

Just as they give rise to new forms of solidarity, lies also produce the
grounds for social exclusion. HIV-positive women are frequently the targets
of lies. Rumors about Mercy's character provided a clear illustration of
this. These insinuations were products of "smoke and mirrors" – elaborate
displays in which people state misleading or irrelevant information to
manipulate others' perceptions. Her relatives' gossip allowed her husband's misdeeds to go unquestioned. Such deceitful statements and
actions effectively silence women, even when they know the truth.

This chapter has questioned what is at stake in women's HIV disclosure.
How do these individuals, disempowered by both the stigma surrounding
their illness and their status as women, maintain their dignity through
speech? They do so, I argued, by managing how, when, and to whom they

share their own and others' positive diagnoses. Laraba, Mercy, and Halima's disclosures occurred in contexts in which they could emphasize their concern for family. In situations where people may question their honor, they hide their condition. Women's respectability is performed through displays of self-care, work, and responsible wifehood and parenthood. At the same time, women must navigate religious and kinship expectations, as well as acute economic needs and obligations. In making these choices, they risk divorce, ill health, HIV transmission, and the loss of their children and possessions. They negotiate these ethical dilemmas through the manipulation of speech. In the next chapter, women use not only speech to present themselves as ethical subjects but also their bodies.

Intimate Ethics

In 2006, I sat in a counseling office at an HIV clinic with Patience, a close friend and key informant. She had worked there for a year as a treatment support specialist. Her day-to-day activities consisted of escorting patients from the lab to the physician's office to the pharmacy. Patience complained that the medical director had asked her to provide guidance on "living positively" to a distraught patient. They hoped Patience would share her personal experiences with her. Although some of the staff members knew she was HIV-positive, many of her clients did not. The hospital policies did not require her to disclose her status, and she resented being asked to do so.

Like many other patients, this young woman believed that her life was over. Patience confronted the client. She said, "Look at my face. Do you know if I am positive or negative?" The woman said she thought she was negative. She continued, "How do you know this?" The woman responded that it was because she was so fat. "In fact," Patience countered, "I am positive . . . so you see, you can live healthy just like everyone, as long as you take your medicine every day." The medical lesson was clear: if you adhere to your treatment regimen, you will remain healthy. However, Patience also imparted to her client a social lesson implicitly understood by all of the women in that clinic's waiting room: beauty – displayed through a curvy, well-dressed body and modest, yet self-assured, comportment – is deceptive.

The medical director hired Patience, in part, because of her HIV status.[1] Although disclosure was not mandatory, this job, in effect, situated

Patience as the "face of HIV" in the clinic. While not explicitly stated to her, Patience needed to be especially attentive to her own health. If she stopped taking drugs or suffered from a series of debilitating chronic illnesses, she thought she would be fired. Then, Patience had been experiencing shooting pains all over her body. Despite taking unpaid leaves to visit specialists and purchase expensive medications, she never received a diagnosis. Patience did not tell the director about the severity of her pain. I suspected this had to do with her fear of jeopardizing her employment status.

Patience's position required more than sustained good health, however. In the clinic, her coworkers and clients regularly remarked upon her appearance. At the time of our discussion, she had recently remarried. When women marry, their physical appearances often change. Patience gained weight, and she now paid greater attention to her clothes, hair, and sense of style. In short, she embodied not only a healthy patient and worker but also a virtuous, married woman.

Because of the disease's physiological effects on the body and its stigma, HIV-positive women often question taken-for-granted assumptions about their gendered identities, including notions of virtue, kinship, and the body. The physical and social threats related to HIV's stigma force women to take inventory of their moral and social resources. In other words, a positive diagnosis also brings to light their ethical sensibilities – that is, the tacit thoughts, actions, and statements that guide them in their efforts to live a good life.

In northern Nigeria, HIV-positive women were especially concerned with how the disease would affect their ability to experience intimacy. Intimacy entails more than sexual acts; it has material, affective, psychological, and physiological dimensions. These women, I observed, work on different aspects of their selves – including their sense of well-being and their close relationships – to produce intimacy in their lives. These diverse activities fit within a larger category of labor called *care work*. This term applies to the efforts people devote to caring for their own and others' bodies. In northern Nigeria, I have found that this labor also includes the cultivation of intimate experience with men, the creation of new and reliable modes of subsistence, the formation of resilient exchange relationships, and, finally, the mending and maintenance of reputations.[2]

For HIV-positive women, these efforts are particularly crucial to their well-being. They offer a response to an array of dilemmas, including the following: What do I do if my husband is unfaithful to me? What if I love someone else? If my husband cannot support our family, what is my responsibility? How can I gain greater power in my household without alienating others? Can I have a baby, even if my husband does not want it? In this chapter's cases, I focus on how these social and ethical quandaries intersect with women's desires, bodies, and exchanges.

BINTA

In the spring of 2007, my friend Rashida and I meandered through one of the narrow paths inside the old city of Kano looking for Binta's house. I had interviewed Binta a number of times earlier that year. She was one of the Muslim HIV-positive widows in the support group I attended. Binta told me her baby was ill when we spoke over the phone and she asked if we could visit her at her home. Like most of the corridors through the old city, an open sewer ran alongside the road. Garbage clogged the conduits. High clay walls plastered with torn, faded posters hid the social activities unfolding in residences behind them.

At the end of one of these routes, we spotted the door to Binta's apartment. We entered and greeted, *salama aleikum*, as we passed through the doorway. A young child said back, *aleikum salaam*. We followed her down a dark hallway of crumbling bricks and dirt. On the left, we saw the entrance to an empty room under renovation. That room belonged to Binta. She could not convince the owners of the house to complete the job. Instead, she shared another room with her son and one of the ten other tenants.

Binta eagerly introduced Rashida and me to the landlord and the other residents. They warmly welcomed us with food and drinks. That afternoon, we lay across her bed and shared the oranges I brought with me, as well as the food her landlord had prepared. We discussed her son's illness. Despite the baby's chubby body, his deep cough and fever made me worry. I did not know his HIV status. Binta, too, was very thin with the same terrible cough. She spoke with a hoarse, cracking voice. I remember leaving her place that day concerned that they were both in far worse shape than Binta would tell us.

When I returned a year and a half later, much to my surprise, Binta had remarried. She looked healthier and happier than she had been in our previous visit. Binta opened the door to her new apartment and let us inside. We followed her into a small but sparkling clean parlor. Thick drapes covered the windows. An ornate hutch stood against one of walls. Its shelves held traditional porcelain dishes and other decorative objects. Although relatively modest, the presence of these items signified a set of successful transactions from Binta's engagement and subsequent wedding. She had told me previously that, in order to continue her business, she had to sell all of the furniture she received from her wedding to her first husband.

Binta appeared content with her new home and her return to married life. That day, she wore a bright yellow blazer and long black skirt. A small hijab covered her hair. Although still petite, she had gained a considerable amount of weight since we last met. Binta smiled throughout our interview. Her beautiful body and her neat, well-furnished home vividly displayed her status as a new bride (*amarya*).

I went to see Binta then to learn more about her experience as a businesswoman in Kano. Thinking back on our conversation a year before, I wanted to know how women like Binta were able to meet their health care, family, and personal needs when they had no one to support them. With limited access to salaried employment in Kano's formal economy, many women generate incomes through their own entrepreneurial activities. Nearly all of the HIV-positive women I interviewed referenced their bodies as vital to their ability to earn and save money. Binta was widely recognized in the support group as a skilled saleswoman.

I began our interview by asking Binta about her work history. She told me that when she was young, she learned how to start a business from her grandparents, who prepared medicinal herbs. They taught her everything she knew. Binta then started to produce and sell herbal treatments for different kinds of bodily issues: fertility problems, bleeding, pregnancy and delivery, sex, and sexually transmitted infections, among others. Binta said that she would go to Kano's major hospitals and sell these remedies to patients and medical staff. Although not employed by a hospital, patients' families would call on her to discuss specific health matters and recommend treatments.

Binta's occupation could be classified as care work, as it involves attending to the bodily, emotional, and sensual needs of other people. Care work may be compensated, in roles such as health care services, household help, or sex work, or uncompensated – including the reproductive and other domestic obligations women must meet. In both compensated and uncompensated roles, women's bodies are essential to this work. Like Patience, who provided intimate details about her life to her clients in order to earn her salary, Binta's body was also central to her success in her herb-selling business.

Binta not only sold medicinal items but also provided valuable information about her personal experience using her treatments. Many conservative Muslims in northern Nigeria would not approve of this work. They would consider it to be dangerous, indecent, or inappropriate for women.[3] For one, it required Binta to move independently around the city, outside of the watchful eyes of her relatives. Of greater concern, as part of her job, Binta engaged in deeply intimate conversations about issues of sexual and reproductive health with strangers, including men. When I asked others about their moral objections, they explained to me that Binta might become too familiar with men and their sexual needs, either seducing them or being seduced into a relationship. This business sustained Binta through her first marriage, as well as the period that followed her husband's death. She knew, nevertheless, that her new husband would dislike or even forbid her from pursuing this work.

Mindful about the need to protect her health and reputation in this marriage, Binta changed occupations. She then began to buy used clothes and sell them to her friends, neighbors, and other customers. As we sat on her couch that afternoon, Binta brought over a pile of carefully folded clothes for me to admire and – she hoped – to purchase. I remarked that there are many women across Kano, as well as many markets, where women conduct this business. I asked her how she found her clientele. What makes her so successful when there is so much competition?

Binta answered, "If I get money, I buy clothes. Then, I sell them on credit – on two installment payments in a month. That is, this month I will be given half and next month I will be given half. . . . I sell fashion, necklaces and earrings, as well as lipsticks. I bring them home and people admire them. If we go to weddings or naming ceremonies, I sell them . . . people tell me, 'Bring it. Let's see.' If it is in hospitals that people need items, I also sell them there."

Binta explained that she wears the clothing that she purchases from these markets, and when women admire her dress, she says she is willing to sell it to them. Or, she added, she could bring similar items if they are interested. For Binta, her beauty not only served to attract admirers, including her doting husband, but also attracted customers. To be successful in this business, Binta had to project an image of a professional, successful, and alluring individual, one who women want to become, in order to create a demand for her goods – in other words, imaginatively rendering herself into an object to be bought and sold.

To describe this kind of labor in a different way, Binta profited from women's need to become desirable to others – namely, men. As in her previous sales position, Binta relied on her body – actually selling the clothes off her back – to generate income. She appeared to be doing very well in her new venture. Binta was only slightly disappointed when the clothes she brought to me did not fit.

Our conversation shifted to her recent marriage. I asked her why she needed to marry another husband. Binta explained:

> I got married because I got tired of suffering and looking for food. Now, sometimes my husband brings, and sometimes I will bring food. If he has money, I will not do it. I married him, however, because of his piety, not because of his money. . . . He is very patient and he has pity. When it is early morning and he gets up, he will not go out until he has asked me, "Did you wake up well? I hope there is not a problem?" If I come back home and he sees that I am tired, he will prepare food for me. I even taught my husband how to cook!

Binta first referenced here the powerlessness and humiliation HIV-positive women feel when they are left alone without husbands to meet even their most basic needs. The ignominy of being unmarried compounds and even surpasses the indignities that accompany life in poverty. Although Binta's current husband could not always economically support her, she appreciated the psychological and spiritual support he provided.

In Binta's description, she explained how her husband would conspicuously display his concern for her health, as well as the well-being of her child – a child who he did not, in fact, father. By cooking dinner, a responsibility that almost always falls on the wife in northern Nigeria, he accomplished two things that Binta valued: first, he paid attention to her body, noting her fatigue or stress, and attempted to relieve her. Second, by occasionally taking on a distinctly feminine domestic chore, her husband allowed Binta to continue to work and avail herself of the benefits that her autonomy and income provided. In contrast with older generations of women, many of the young women I knew stated that their ideals of marital intimacy included the mutual exchange of emotional and material care. These relationships still hinged on the condition of their bodies, however.

Binta contemplated a dilemma faced by many working women: How do you mask your husband's inability to fulfill these economic expectations and protect him (as well as yourself) from this shame? And, while safeguarding his reputation, how do you maintain your respectability and independence in your own work?[4] This is a particularly important concern for Binta given that communities and families closely monitor women's roles in the workforce for signs of impropriety. For men, the inability to support your family exposes your dishonorable character. Married women typically feel morally obliged to keep their husbands' shortcomings secret.

These social stakes are even higher when a woman and her partner must keep others from suspecting they live with HIV. Vacillating between the value of work and her gendered moral principles, Binta elaborated:

> Before, my problems were too many. Now I purchase food with his money, even if I do not work. I will still work once in a while, since his salary is not much. If his money finishes (runs out), that is when you will see me suffer a little. If he is getting a little money, even if the food is not delicious, we will still eat. He has lessened my suffering. Prior to this marriage, when I had to go out to work, I was thin and even lighter than you. Now, if he gets a good job and I do not have to go out, I intend to become beautiful and fat. But you see, sometimes, if he does not have money, I go out to look for a hundred or fifty naira. He does not stop me because he does not want me to owe. If you see a man stopping his wife from working, it is because he has taken away all her responsibilities. He satisfies her desires. . . . If he cannot take away her needs and he trusts her, he can allow her to go out. My husband does not have the power to help me. You see, all my brothers' responsibilities are on my head. (I must help out my brothers). . . . If I make a profit, it is mine, and I can buy more with this capital. It is better than going to the street to beg for alms or pleading with others to help me. I was humiliating myself before. God has not stopped me from looking for money, so long as the work is not sinful.

On one hand, Binta felt grateful that her husband allowed her to work. This enabled her, in turn, to contribute to their household expenses and to meet her obligations to others. On the other hand, if her husband had a good job, she would not need to work and her appearance would improve. Although not stated explicitly, if Binta's looks improved, her HIV status would remain concealed. Her beauty would also keep her husband's attention. This might stop him from pursuing extramarital relationships. Binta could also rely on her body to enhance her business, if she needed to return to work in the future.

Some northern Nigerians would argue that a husband who extends his permission for his wife to work does so because he lacks concern for her reputation. Others might say his decision reflects his own laziness or ineptitude in securing employment. To me, Binta appeared to suggest that her husband's permission was not a result of his moral faults but rather his concern that she should not owe money to others. Although poverty itself is indeed humiliating, in Binta's mind, women's indebtedness to others is a greater offense.

In northern Nigeria, poverty and debt go hand in hand. Most poor and working-class women cannot access credit through financial institutions or other formal channels. Commonly, they incur debts with people who they see on a regular basis. And, when women owe others, they attempt to avoid them until they have the money to repay their loans. Debt thus forces people into undesirable face-to-face confrontations. If these obligations become publicly known, they may raise questions over a woman's character or the circumstances of her marriage and family life: How is she spending her money? Why don't her parents or husband support her?

For HIV-positive women, their debts may poison the very relationships that they worked so hard to forge and protect. The unpredictable and uncontrollable social repercussions from a soured exchange could pose a significant threat to their well-being. HIV-positive women fear that people will say these moral failings show proof of their blameworthiness for their infection. Debt is thus a particularly risky venture. To avoid debt altogether, a woman must possess substantial economic and social capital. In this last passage, Binta made the connection directly. Although they are poor, her husband's permission to work provides her a privilege that many other women do not possess.

To demonstrate her virtue, Binta not only worked to eschew debt but also sought to selflessly and generously support others. As we ended the interview, she explained to me that she felt closer to God by living with her neighbors peacefully and giving alms (*zakat*). I was surprised to hear Binta emphasize this obligation, given her modest income. From her description, however, I realized that almsgiving was a way to display her consideration for her neighbors and friends. Binta continued: "If I have good things, I share them with people. When we were in (my former) house, we were ten in number. If I went off to do some business, whatever sweet item I would get while out, I would cook it. Then, I would show it off and give it to everyone. If they collect it from me and eat it, I will get a reward."

When Binta's first husband fell sick, she feared that no one would come to check on him or offer her assistance if they knew his status. She said she would not be able to live in peace without friends to visit. If she gives generously, beyond what her family and friends typically expect from her, she hopes they will repay her in the form of emotional, social, or material support when she eventually will need it. Binta's point reminded me of the generous reception I received in her former house, despite signs indicating she was not doing well. When I returned this visit, I gave her a small gift of perfume, which pleased her. From Binta's perspective, I think that this series of exchanges and hospitable gestures cemented our relationship, not only as researcher and subject but also as a friend and potential business connection.

Binta's narrative reveals central themes critical to understanding the relationship between intimacy and the ethical dilemmas HIV-positive women face as they live healthy lives with a deeply stigmatizing virus. She provided insight into the role women's bodies play in their efforts to earn money. Her case also hinted at some of the hazards of care work occupations, such as the threats a sickly, unattractive body pose to business or the immoral reputation a woman might acquire if she becomes *too* familiar with a client's intimate needs. She also raised questions about the uncompensated kinds of care men and women offer one another in the domestic sphere. Binta quickly learned that her new husband could not entirely meet their household needs. Her business success masked her husband's inability to support their family. Furthermore, a stable income mitigated the risk that visible displays of poverty would expose her status to the public. Binta's work also allowed her to share her earnings with others. These investments complemented her efforts to build a support network that will benefit them in the future.

ROSE

In 2010, I conducted an interview with Rose, a thirty-one-year-old Christian from Kaduna State. We met in a large, private conference room that served as the meeting space for their monthly HIV support group meeting. It was located off a long corridor, away from the crowded waiting area at the main entrance of the hospital. In the mornings, nurses occasionally used the space to change from their clothes into their uniforms. Over the course of the day, some of the Muslim women on the hospital staff would enter and pray in a quiet corner of the room. At four o'clock or so in the afternoons, the women returned to the room to change back into their regular clothes. They chatted with one another while they tied their wrappers, reapplied their makeup, and adjusted their veils. I found this congenial and distinctly gendered space a good setting for my interviews. That visit, I focused on women's beauty regimens and the ways in which they give and receive different kinds of help.

Rose looked much like many of the well-dressed women in the waiting room that day. She wore tight pants and a stylish blouse, and her hair was intricately braided. Although she was a Christian, she had a small, translucent veil carelessly draped over her head. Rose quickly removed the veil once seated. Rashida, my research assistant, flashed me a knowing smile. Rose's appearance suggested to us that she possessed a sensibility about beauty, which we had witnessed over and over in the clinic. I asked her bluntly what her thoughts were on women's beauty.

Rose answered, "Beauty always . . . well, you need to bathe, be neat, and wear makeup." I pressed, "What type of makeup?" Rose listed, "Brush your teeth, apply eye shadow, shape your eyebrows, rub powder, use eye pencil, paint your mouth, and plait your hair very fine . . . or wash your hair. I normally shape my eyebrows in the market."

I probed further: "You mean it is only your face and hair that makes you beautiful? No other part of the body?" "No," Rose said. "You buy nice clothes, you wear perfume. . . ." As she trailed off, I continued, "So tell us, what does a well-dressed woman, like you, wear?"

> On weekdays, you wear trousers, skirts, and small tops. Then, on Sundays, when I go to church, I wear wrappers (traditional cloth), or lace or Holland (an expensive brand of traditional cloth) – anything that I can tie and appear mature, like a married woman. Married women tie wrappers and use big head ties. Like today, I am coming here from school, so I am wearing trousers and a top. . . . You also bathe three times a day. Change your underclothes, especially your underwear. You should not wear the same pair from morning until evening because of the heat . . . unless you are not at home. But then, even if you are at your working place, there is a bathroom. You could bathe and change there. Men are always looking at you on the street. You also have to dress well at home. And, you have to clean your house very well because of visitors.

Rose's efforts to care for her body were not exceptional among northern Nigerian women. To add to this catalog of daily practices, other women listed traditional perfumes and roll-on (deodorants), earrings, bangles, necklaces, hijabs and veils, henna design on hands and feet, lipstick, eyelash extensions, and straightening or relaxing one's hair. Women also named styles of clothes ranging from designer European and American brands to dresses, tops, and skirts made out of expensive traditional West African fabrics (Holland and English wax cloth and Swiss laces, among others), lingerie, nightgowns, shoes, and matching handbags. HIV-positive women would prominently and even proudly display these beauty items and practices.

Although these practices vary between Muslims and Christians, women uniformly stated that they must invest in their appearances. Rose said that she earned the money to pay for these beauty products and clothes by preparing pepper soup in another woman's restaurant. She explained that she would sell as much as 20,000 Naira ($125) of meat in a day, as well as would clean the restaurant. Rose added that if she did not maintain a neat appearance, customers would not come. The care she devoted to her living environment, in other words, was an extension of her beauty and crucial to her livelihood, just as it was for Binta.

"If you take your medications, eat well, keep your surroundings clean, and keep your body neat, people will never know about your status?" I asked. She replied, "Just eat good food that will give you protein. Sometimes, when I have money, I buy some fruits. I buy malt drinks. Nobody knows that I have HIV. . . . (But, if you wear clothes that are not pretty) they will suspect you. Maybe you are sick, or you suffer from a mental illness, or you are a dirty woman. There is nothing they cannot say. But if you come out appearing neat, no one will suspect you."

In these detailed descriptions of women's beauty regimens, Rose emphasized themes consistent across many of my discussions with HIV-positive women. Like all women, those who live with HIV navigate social dilemmas with and through their bodies. They accentuate some features while they hide others.

Through her body, Rose documented how she would fend off any suspicion of HIV, while at the same time defying popular pronouncements regarding people with AIDS living at the site of a grave (*kabari kusa*). However, I think Rose was also doing much more than that. HIV-positive women dress well not merely to attract the interest or secure the respect of men who pass by them on the street. They also aim to present an outward image of people they want to become – namely, virtuous, married, and respectable women. Bodily practices provide women ways of shaping their futures.[5]

While I initially thought she was just listing products, activities, and features that enhanced a woman's attractiveness, I soon learned that Rose's body was at the forefront of her thoughts as she contemplated a much larger dilemma: her marriage, at the time of our interview, was in the process of disintegrating. She felt torn between a husband who knew her status but maltreated her and an old boyfriend, who loved her and would give her money and advice. Rose's vigilant attention to her appearance was a means of keeping her status hidden while she figured out what to do about her relationship.

Rose's current interest, Peter, was her first true love. She met him in her family's village in Kaduna. She described to me the first time he saw her:

> Then, I was twelve years old. I went to the market to buy something. A young man stopped me on the way and said I was beautiful. When he said it, I told him to leave me alone. . . . I wanted to pass, but then he would stop me. If I turned to the other side, he would stop me again. When I laughed, he said, "See, your open teeth!" (a gap in her teeth). I did not know about open teeth at that time. It was not until I came to Kano and became a bit

civilized (that I realized what he was referring to and why he was flirting with me).

Shortly after, his father died and his family sent him to Lagos to live with relatives. They lost touch. Rose had a number of other boyfriends while in school. When she moved to Kano to stay with her relatives, she had her first sexual relationship. I asked her what it was like, and she elaborated, "We would always hold hands and walk together. We always felt like kissing each other. We held each other and romanced each other. Sometimes, from romance, we would then go to bed together." As she gave these accounts of her early relationships, her bodily experience was at the center of her descriptions of intimacy.

Eventually, Rose met the man she would marry. They had a sexual relationship for nearly five years before deciding to wed. The reverend father in their church told them that they must go for an HIV test. Although she had never been sick, Rose tested HIV positive. Her fiancé was negative. "What happened?" I wanted to know.

> I started crying. The doctor comforted me and told me not to cry. It was not the end of my life. Then, we went to the reverend and told him the result. He asked, "What kind of problem is it? Pregnancy?" I told him that I was HIV-positive. He asked about my husband. I said that he was negative. From there, I told my husband the truth. I told him I would not force him to marry me because I do not want him to run away from me tomorrow.

When she met with her reverend, she discussed her fears with him. Rose reiterated to him that she did not want her husband to reject her at some point in the future. She thought he would harass or leave her because he did not have the virus and she did. Her husband, however, still wanted to marry her.

Despite her concerns, the reverend encouraged them to proceed. His response, in effect, was, "Who are you, the HIV-positive woman, to turn down a man who agrees to marry you?" Although Rose did not say this explicitly, I believe she understood him to mean that he did not think it likely she would ever find a husband because of her HIV status. In their different visions of the future, Rose's infection was at the center of this dilemma: she believed her status would eventually ignite conflicts with her husband, while her reverend imagined a future where she would be relegated to life as an unmarriageable woman. These assumptions were common among many of the men and women I met, both HIV-positive and HIV-negative.

I asked Rose later in our discussion whether she was afraid her husband would tell others about her status. She insisted, "If he says it, it does not concern me because I did not buy [HIV] in the market. I did not willingly bring it upon myself. . . . If I got it through sex, my husband too would have caught it. Because I was with him for years before we even got married."

Put another way, if he sought to expose her status to the public, Rose felt she had proof that she could not have contracted the virus from sex. Her husband was not infected, and he was her only sexual partner for the five years that preceded her marriage. Rose thought that her husband, then, could not accuse her of immoral sexual behavior.

Even so, Rose was upfront in the beginning of our interview that she did not tell anyone, other than her reverend, about her test result. She did not want anyone to know. On one hand, a healthy husband could defend her from others' suspicions. On the other, her husband possessed the power to discredit her character if he chose to tell people. Given the negligible amount of power she had in the relationship, the condition of her own body became even more crucial.

Rose and her husband must not only remain healthy, she said. They must also present an image of virtue and prosperity. She cannot alienate her husband or provoke his anger, or she risks destabilizing an already precarious relationship. I found it noteworthy that she left out the fact that her husband would, in all likelihood, be reluctant to tell anyone her status – angry or not. It would cast public suspicion on their relationship. If other women learned he had a wife of five years who was HIV-positive, they would undoubtedly suspect him of lying about his status.

Just three days before the wedding, Rose's first boyfriend, who she had not heard from since she was twelve years old, called her. "That day, my phone rang. The man said his name was Peter, but I could not place it. He then described himself. I screamed and asked him if he was still alive. He said, 'Yes! . . . I saw your invitation, so I decided to surprise you with this call.'"

Over the phone that day, they talked about the wedding, and he advised her to "think very well. Marriage is not a day job." She considered his advice and wanted to run away from the wedding. Another close friend cautioned her not to do it. Although she was unhappy, Rose went through with the marriage. "It was not easy," she recalled.

From the beginning, the marriage was fraught with problems. For the first few months, things were fine, Rose stressed. They would pray together and her husband's salary increased. But then, inexplicably, he stopped sleeping at home and would only return to her in the mornings. He would not give her money for her food or clothes. After more than a year of this economic neglect, he then began to ignore her entirely. Finally, Rose gave in. She woke her husband in the middle of the night to ask him what was wrong. She said, "Even if I offended you, tell me, and I will ask for your forgiveness." He told her to stop disturbing him.

Soon after, her husband proclaimed that he was giving her twenty-four hours to pack and leave his house. Rose refused. She said that she was not going anywhere. He then left her and moved into a friend's house, effectively abandoning her entirely. Rose continued, "If he wants me to return to my parents, he should take me to the reverend who married us first. I told him he has to say all he has to say to me in the presence of the reverend father." Her husband rebuffed this request. At the time of our interview, she had not heard from him in over two months.

Patience, the counselor, was her close friend. I asked Rose if she sought her advice. She nodded and answered:

I told her my husband ran away. She said I should continue praying that one day God will bring an end to this sickness. "Nothing that has a beginning does not also have an end." I should take care of myself and eat well, bathe, and not think about it. She said they would also put me in their prayers. As always, if I feel any pains whatsoever I should rush to the hospital. But, it is like these drugs cost money. . . . The little money that God gives me, I manage to buy food, soap, plait my hair, and keep myself neat. Because I cannot say to others, "Give me something."

"Why not?" I asked.

In Nigeria you can't go begging people. If you say, "Give me . . ." after you leave them, they will start gossiping about you. You better fight for your own. If you keep begging, they will call you a beggar . . . that is why . . . if you see how I suffer [at work], I do not care. Because, I know that by the month's end I will have a small amount of money to use to solve my problems.

The core of the advice Rose received from Patience was the need for her to continue to take care of her body.[6] She can then produce a different future for herself – one in which HIV will not be the end of her life. Patience's advice articulated a culturally specific notion of well-being (*lafiya*), which is situated in a constellation of elements, including both the personal and the communal, safety and beauty, and networks of reciprocity and social relations.

To some extent, Rose subscribed to this endeavor; however, her thoughts almost immediately turned back to the economic cost of this set of practices. Medical care, in particular, is expensive. Although they have access to subsidized HIV medications, patients must still pay to treat other illnesses – some associated with the virus and others that are unrelated, but part of a set of chronic disorders from which Nigerians routinely suffer.

Rose ended her discussion with me by reiterating her hope that her husband would allow their relationship just to end. She would then be free to marry someone else. During her marriage, Rose had reacquainted with Peter. He flirted with her and gave her money when she needed it. "So that was why we are waiting for him," she said, indirectly referring to her wish that Peter marry her.

In the meantime, Rose was taking his advice to concentrate on her education and career. "I cannot leave my current marriage and jump into another fire. I have to rest and relax." In the space between the present, in which women face seemingly unrelenting suffering, and the future, where their hopes for a better life lie, they must be patient and focus on things within their control. Rose's body, her friendship with Peter, and her education were at the center of her efforts to pass the time in a meaningful way.

Rose's narrative expanded on Binta's descriptions of the roles that women's bodies play in navigating their social dilemmas, financial needs, and intimate desires. Specifically, Rose's conspicuous beauty hints at how bodies provide women a palette for expressing both their social status and their aspirations for the future.[7] She highlighted how the cleanliness of her workplace was an extension of her beauty practices and how necessary beauty and hygiene were to securing employment, attracting customers, and earning an income. Women's orientations toward the future, Rose demonstrated, shape the way they think about and work upon their bodies.

TALATU

Talatu was forty years old and a Christian, originally from Adamawa State, in the northeastern region of the country. She identified her ethnicity as both Hausa and Babur. Talatu had been married to a man for fourteen years. He was also HIV-positive. She gave birth to six children over the course of her married life, three of whom are still alive. Talatu's first baby died at delivery in breech position. The oldest was thirteen, the middle child was ten, and the youngest was a two-year-old girl. Prior to her baby girl, she had given birth to two boys with developmental disabilities who died at young ages. Talatu told me in the beginning of our first interview that she had recently conceived again but had yet to tell her husband.

Although she had many suitors when she was young, Talatu finally met the man she would marry at a church event in Katsina State. She was then twenty-four. He was from Jos, where Talatu also lived at the time. About two years after their first meeting, they finally wed. Initially the marriage was good, Talatu said. They spoke freely and lovingly to each other. They never quarreled. "Anything you want," she elaborated, "he would give it. Food, water, clothes, everything." Her husband never complained or said that the things she wanted cost too much.

Talatu, in turn, was also devoted to him. She told me how she would change her dress in the morning and evening each day, so that he would not see her in the same clothes twice. Talatu wore makeup daily and plaited her hair because she knew he admired her face and hair, in particular. Like Rose, she was attentive to her hygiene as well as the condition of their house. She cleaned constantly. Her mother and siblings had advised her on how to take care of him.

Echoing a theme raised by many of the women with whom I spoke, Talatu said, "If you do not do these things, you will lose your husband's attention. He will be looking at others outside." Acts of adultery, women in Talatu's support group argued, are unambiguously immoral. And yet, they are also intertwined with men's natural sexual instincts. Another member added, "We women could see a neat, good-looking man, but not be moved. Men, however, would not hesitate to follow a well-dressed woman, even though he is knowledgeable, informed, and might have just finished preaching in the mosque. He will see and follow a woman. That is why we keep seeing all sorts of problems in our lives."

Men, according to many northern Nigerian women, innately need more sex than women. Hauwa, another member of the support group, expanded on this. She said that infidelity is due to wives being "dirty, unfaithful, and not looking after herself properly. . . . If the man comes to her and finds her smelly and the bed un-welcoming, he tends to be drawn to someone else who is neat, and looks and smells nice." Northern Nigerian women who cannot appear beautiful, neat, and "cultured" risk losing their husbands to "outside women."

To meet these virtuous ideals, however, wives must possess material resources, which, not coincidentally, men are responsible for providing. Husbands who neglect their wives, potentially leading to their unkempt appearance, then feel justified in pursuing new girlfriends. At the same time, women blame themselves for their lack of "culture," when it is, in fact, larger inequalities out of their control driving these betrayals.

I asked Talatu how, if at all, things changed after being married for so long. "How do you keep your husband interested in you?" She emphasized again that both her manner of speaking and her appearance were critical:

> There are times that he will come to the house and is angry. Even when he speaks, I do not respond angrily or answer him back. I speak to him quietly and politely. This has helped me a lot. And, even when he comes back home, he does not see a dirty house. Before he comes back, I take care of the children and myself. . . . Beauty also matters a lot. Now, it is because he is not around (staying at our home in Kano) that my hair is not plaited. But, before he comes, I will plait it because I know he will complain.

Talatu referenced here a wide range of activities that constitute the different kinds of care a woman must provide her husband. These include the maintenance of personal and domestic hygiene, the provision of sensual and sexual pleasure, meeting reproductive needs, and the ability to mollify her husband's emotions and bolster his sense of masculinity. Talatu relied heavily on her body to attend to these demands and desires. But she valued her ability to reason with her husband the most. Nearly all women identified "speaking well" as a trait that exemplifies their beauty and character.

As the marriage progressed, Talatu learned that her husband came from a family that did not respect women's opinions or choices. She raised her voice in our discussion when she informed me that this was one of the things he hid from her before they married. Talatu resented being powerless to challenge her husband. He went to his mother to ask her advice but would not consult with Talatu about these same matters. Her in-laws disliked her, Talatu explained. They even attempted to arrange another marriage for their son. Although they were not ultimately successful, she did not trust them.

Not long after the in-laws' failed intervention, problems surfaced in their marriage. In addition to hiding his money and refusing to pay for household expenses, her husband stopped telling her where he would go in the evenings. She learned about his affairs from his friends. Talatu claimed that she never told her husband that she knew about them. She would, however, let him know when one of his girlfriends came by the house to greet him just to see how he would respond. His face gave it away, Talatu noted. He would also pick fights with her, even when she did nothing wrong. She seemed to take for granted that she should not confront her husband. In fact, Talatu implied she was obliged to protect his secret.

Talatu would not elaborate on how she contracted HIV in our conversation. She confirmed that her husband too was HIV-positive and he blamed her for bringing the virus into their family. Talatu was the first to receive the test. After hearing about this series of deceptions and what seemed to me to be an unfair accusation, I expected Talatu to be angry, yet she spoke matter-of-factly, perhaps suggesting that this provocation was not unusual.

Talatu also continued to have admirers pursue her after her marriage, although she claimed they were not sexual relationships. She realized early on that she had too much to lose if her husband learned about the attention she received from men – even if she just meant to make him jealous. Talatu explained, "Once, there was somebody who approached me when I was working in the company. He said that he was in love with me. So, I told my husband about him and he said I should stop working there because if he ever sees me with another man, it means that I have consented to the affair."

After her husband threatened to make her leave her job, Talatu stopped telling him about these men. She continued, however, to accept their money. "If I am given money, I collect it. . . . If I tell my husband about a gift or money that someone gave me, he would be angry and say that the man wants to have a relationship with me. So, I do not tell him, even if it means lying and saying that I bought the things myself."

Gifts of money and other items in Nigeria communicate a number of things; for example, they demonstrate men's wealth, independence, and their "modern" identities.[8] Even after women marry, admirers often continue to play a role in this gift economy. Men may give expensive gifts and money in exchange for sex. Or, they may simply offer women money to remind them that they admire or appreciate them.

For women who receive little or no economic support from their husbands, these exchanges may supplement their meager earnings. In a context where men frequently abandon, divorce, or widow their wives while they are still in their reproductive years, women know that they will likely remarry in the future. One of the women with whom I worked said that first marriages are usually the parents' choice, while second marriages are for love. Such comments helped me understand better why Rose cared so much about her boyfriend, despite her marriage to another man.

Talatu's conflict with her husband intensified around the same time that they learned their HIV status. It occurred soon after the death of their two sons. Talatu threw herself even more intensely into the work of taking care of the household and her children. She spent the money she earned to cover expenses her husband did not provide. Although married women are not expected to have many, if any, economic responsibilities in their homes, wives may buy their own clothing or help with groceries. "Sometimes wives just do it because they want to," Talatu reasoned.

Talatu and I went through the list of these household expenses: rent ("He is the one that does that. But at times, maybe, I might give some to complete it."), food ("Well, he helps, he provides, but I also help in that aspect too."), and cosmetics and clothes ("At times, he does that, but I also do. . . . And some clothes, if I see and admire them, I buy. Or, even if it's for the children, I buy without even telling him.").

I asked Talatu who spent more money on the household and she stated adamantly that she provided much more than her husband. Despite her insistence that she helped out with these expenses out of her own volition, her efforts stood in contrast with cultural expectations that husbands meet these responsibilities. In nearly all of my conversations with women about money, they mentioned contradictions between religious and cultural ideals and the realities of their investments.

Talatu's efforts to help others extended well beyond the support she devoted to her husband and children. For example, she would often visit her parents, who lived far away from Kano. In addition to paying for the transportation costs, she would bring them food or tea items, among other goods. Talatu would also help her siblings when she could. If they needed help with school fees for their children, she would give it to them. When her sister marries, she said, the cost of the wedding will be split among the family members, including herself. Likewise, Talatu regularly purchased wedding gifts for her friends, such as shoes, bags, or a necklace, and money on the wedding day. Because she had a somewhat stable income from her teaching position, family members continually asked her for loans. Talatu gave whatever she could.

Talatu was equally committed to assisting her neighbors, even if they did not ask her directly. She told me:

> Neighbors, at times, require a lot of help. There are some who . . . maybe if someone died, you should go to the house and offer your condolences. Then you should give something to them, like money. Or cook food and take it to them . . . or even if it is a naming ceremony, if you enter and you give them something, it is also *taimako* (help). Or even maybe, among their children, you notice that the kind of clothes that they wear are tattered, you can put some money aside and buy clothes to give to the family.

Although she did not specify precisely why, I think Talatu would argue that she was simply doing what any pious and respectable woman would do: "because sometimes women just want to help," to echo her earlier comment.

Most women would also readily identify the assistance they give others as a religious virtue. However, Talatu's systematic attention to who is in need of assistance and what they should receive suggested to me that there is more to this virtue than its irreducible moral essence. The help Talatu offers her family and neighbors, in other words, could be read as an extension of who she is as a person and her obligation to the social network within which she is situated. While she did not state this to me in exactly this way, I think she hoped these gestures would make it difficult for her family and neighbors to isolate or abandon her.

Nevertheless, none of these interpretations fully explain the fervency of Talatu's efforts, which were disproportionate to the assistance she received from others. In fact, she claimed, she received almost no support from anyone, apart from the occasional help of her husband and boyfriends. Perhaps because her gestures were *not* being reciprocated or even recognized as worthy of such, they constitute acts of generosity rather than gift exchanges. A gift commonly means a person will return the favor. Talatu's generous gestures thus underline larger structural inequalities.

As we turned to a discussion of Talatu's current problems in her marriage, she began by saying that her husband was frequently out of town. He worked for two weeks at a time in another city. A number of his relatives had recently moved into their house. He had not discussed the arrangement with Talatu, nor did not he provide her with enough money to help pay for the additional expenses of caring for a larger household. Had she known, she would have requested more money from him, Talatu said. She protested to him, but her husband did not worry about how she would care for them. If she refused to pay, they would be suspicious about their marriage. Furthermore, they would gossip about her inability to manage her house. His relatives would assume Talatu was selfishly hoarding the money her husband provided her.

With her in-laws in her house, Talatu faced a dilemma. She explained, "Everything you are eating, you have to give to the others. You cannot separate your own part from theirs." I had asked her earlier about how HIV affected her ability to care for herself. Talatu said:

> Now, I have to really take care of what I eat more than before. Before, you could cook your stew without putting anything in it. But now, you have to add crayfish or some other thing in the stew to make it a bit more nutritious. Then, I also have to eat fruits. And, if you are going to eat it at home, when children are watching you, you cannot isolate yourself. You have to give them some to eat.

To maintain her weight, Talatu must enrich her diet with more expensive foods. And yet, if her children, relatives, or neighbors knew she had these items, she could not hide them. If she did not share, they might ask why she prepares her own special foods separately. This point was reiterated to me by many HIV-positive women.[9]

As another patient described, one of the most obvious signs of an impoverished household was a crying child. She explained that if she went without eating for a day, no one would know. But if someone heard her children constantly crying outside of the house, her neighbors would suspect that her husband did not leave her enough money for food. The same held true for Talatu's relatives, as they would inevitably tell others of their neglect or maltreatment.

Talatu highlighted the demands placed upon her, both as a person infected with HIV and as a woman. Her HIV status rendered her vulnerable to a number of illnesses, which threatened to devalue her body in material, social, and symbolic ways. The disease could rob her of her ability to work, for example. It could also result in the dissolution of her marriage. Consequently, it would discredit her as a wife and a mother.

Given these numerous threats, counselors at the clinic expected others, particularly Talatu's husband or close family members, to take care of her. Talatu, however, did not receive this support. At the same time that HIV placed new restrictions on taken-for-granted bodily practices, such as her diet, she also felt coerced by her husband and his family into giving more of herself – her money, food, time, and labor – to caring for others. This pressure was reinforced by the weight of both cultural expectations and the fact that Talatu had resources available to her from her work as a teacher.

Although Talatu remarked upon the seeming impossibility of this situation, the obligations to feed and care for family were axiomatic truths for most women. While his family members were worthy recipients of these generous acts, Talatu's ardent efforts to give generously to these family members went unacknowledged, unappreciated, or quickly forgotten. Her actions may have been successful in that they masked her HIV status and the potentially larger moral breech of being married to a husband who does not provide for her. Yet, this misrecognition, where her family failed to reciprocate their support in this unspoken exchange expectation, served to undercut the power Talatu desired to attain within her household.

Nevertheless, Talatu continued to emphasize how her income provided her options that she would not otherwise possess. I asked her whether

her husband knew about the money she contributed to her household. She said if he were aware of her investments, he would discourage her from spending her money on the things she felt that she and the children needed. In other words, he wanted to be the one to make the decisions on their household's priorities.

Even though, Talatu pointed out, he did not feel obligated to tell her how he planned to spend his income. He would help his parents and siblings or invest his money in other projects without her consent. In fact, he would not even discuss the matter with her or ask her for advice. Thus, Talatu did not tell her husband about the things for which she was saving until after she had paid for them. This way, he could not say no or tell her to spend her income in a different way. Talatu concluded, "If you do not have money, even if you are the eldest in the family, you become a nobody. Because if, for example, there is a decision that needs to be made, your husband and family will not even ask you for your opinion before making a decision."

I asked another married friend from Kano to explain this to me. "Why would her husband not support her? Would he not be pleased or even grateful to have a wife willing to help, even when she is not obligated to do so?" My friend laughed at me and called this dynamic "the African factor." From her perspective, if a woman contributes a lot of money to the household, she is jostling for power in the marriage. Her money allows her to have more of a say in family matters, as well as the ability to plan for their future, with or without her husband's consent. If a wife refuses to follow her husband's advice, she said, he would blame her defiance on her money. That is why Talatu did not tell her husband how much she makes or the plans she made for her savings.

While Talatu was reluctant to discuss details about her own experience in testing HIV-positive, she eagerly spoke about her recent pregnancy and her children: "You know, a few years ago, before my last girl, I had two boys. But their development was very slow. They were not growing as they should . . . because at the age of one year, one of them was not even sitting up by himself. He suffered many illnesses before he died. That was before I was diagnosed or started taking treatments."

Talatu's two-year-old daughter, however, gave her an enormous amount of pride. She was not only healthy but also intelligent and mature for her age. She could already speak, Talatu exclaimed. She added, "I am teach-ing her some of the rhymes that I teach in school. When you tell her to sing them, she sings! If you tell her to pray before you eat, she prays!" In the face of so many assaults on Talatu's physical body and social status, precipitated by her HIV infection – in addition to the apparent neglect of those who were supposed to support her – childbirth gave Talatu a means of resisting these dominating social forces. By emphasizing her daughter's precocity, she sought to convince me that HIV would not, in fact, keep her from having healthy and smart children.

It was impossible for me to know for sure whether or in what ways HIV affected the health of her two late sons. Because Talatu stressed that the death of her sons took place before she received a test or treatments, I suspect that these events were related in her mind. In short, her healthy daughter was proof that Talatu could fulfill these gendered expectations surrounding motherhood. She felt that her new pregnancy, both sym-bolically and materially, challenged popular notions of the defiling and debilitating effects HIV has on the body. In short, it provided Talatu an embodied sign of her hope for the future.

And yet, Talatu also knew that her husband did not share this opti-mism. She explained further, "Because of the past experience with my two late sons, my husband does not want me to conceive. . . . I am keeping away from him until the time I will come here to confirm that I am pregnant or when he comes to the clinic. He is always saying he does not want me to conceive right now. When he comes back to Kano and the pregnancy is confirmed, then I will let him know." Given his reluctance to have another child, I asked Talatu how she thought her husband would respond to this news. She said, "He will be happy, but he will say I should remove (abort) it. . . . But then, when the child grows up and becomes something, he will say this is his child."

Through our conversation, Talatu weighed what a child could do for her marital relationship with the social risk of her husband learning of her pregnancy too soon. Although she was a few months into her pregnancy, she had yet to seek prenatal care. In northern Nigeria, there remain sig-nificant risks in childbirth, regardless of HIV status. Talatu was willing to assume these risks, or at least seemed uninterested in discussing them with me, because of her desire to have this baby. In addition, Talatu fully expected that her husband would refuse, at least initially, to recognize the child as his own. He would not economically support him or her, just as he refused to provide for her daughter.

Talatu hoped, nonetheless, that her husband's attitude would change once he saw that the child would be healthy like their youngest daughter. Despite her tumultuous reproductive history and the medical risks HIV presents, her conviction was unsurprising given the critical importance of children to a woman's sense of self. Talatu's optimism stemmed from her faith that God would protect their family.

From the vivid and enthusiastic description of her first daughter's behavior, it sounded to me like Talatu conspicuously displayed her daughter's health and development to her husband, hoping to convince him of both of their worth. A new baby might resolve a seemingly intractable situation, in which her husband would not fulfill his symbolic or economic expectations to his family. More important, I think Talatu hoped that a baby would even bring them closer together in their relationship, in which they would exchange respect, appreciation, and even love for one another, not just money.[10]

THE LABOR OF CARE

To secure their well-being, HIV-positive women devote themselves to meeting the bodily, emotional, and sensual needs of others. What makes their acts of care work particularly striking is how heavily they rely on their own bodies to carry out these efforts. For example, Binta and Rose's appearance enticed their customers to spend more money on the goods they sold. Their customers wanted not only clothes and a good meal; they also demanded the services of beautiful women as a necessary part of the value of their purchases. Pleasure, flirtation, admiration, and intimate knowledge are intangible qualities accompanying expectations of these occupations. All three women hoped that these efforts would ultimately result in support from others.

Like their customers and family members, they desired more than just consumable items: Binta, Rose, and Talatu each sought to finance their future aspirations, such as school fees for their children and themselves, costs associated with maintaining beautiful and attractive bodies, and investments in their businesses. Their ventures, they hoped, would enable them to attract caring partners and husbands, to achieve greater autonomy in their households and occupations, and to meet kinship expectations. These moral strivings are at the core of what it means to be a woman.

An HIV-positive diagnosis exposes cracks in the tacit assumptions women possess over how they are expected to live "positively" – or virtuously – as they confront broader social forces that leave them vulnerable to violence, inequality, and poor health. All of these women in this chapter believed that HIV had the potential to symbolically devalue their bodies. This devaluation is compounded by their poverty, neglectful husbands and families, and gendered norms that are constraining, disabling, and seemingly impossible to fully realize. The virus produces a new set of social and health care needs, which often require the assistance – and compassion – of others. And yet, these commitments are difficult to secure as women often feel too ashamed to disclose their status, as well as too embarrassed to beg for help from others.

Nevertheless, this same diagnosis also allows us to understand how women persevere, assert their agency, and reimagine their futures. Specifically, HIV-positive women's commitment to caring for others calls attention to the ways ethics are embedded in intimate experiences. Binta, Talatu, and Rose's experiences offer profound displays of hope in the face of uncertainty, hypocrisy, and injustice. Their stories offer a window into the fact that women can – *and do* – transcend the physiological and social death sentences that too commonly haunt this disease.

Hope

Because of global donors' increasing investment in HIV treatment programs over the past decade, the number of support groups across the country has multiplied exponentially.[1] In Kano city alone, there are at least seven, comprising several hundred HIV-positive men and women. On the wall of one of the offices where I conducted interviews, there was a framed document outlining the vision of the support group. In line with the expectations of these donors, it stated that their central mission was to "promote a self-sufficient society, the alleviation of poverty, and the reduction of stigma." The nongovernmental organizations that sponsor support groups also assist them by serving as venues for programs that address "social care."[2] HIV-positive men and women may access resources, such as legal services, linkages to food support, and income-generating programs, primarily through enrollment and involvement in these groups. In addition, clinicians, public health workers, and researchers, like me, recruit people in these sites for different kinds of studies, interventions, and public events.[3]

In northern Nigeria, however, the actual reasons why men and women joined and benefited from support groups sometimes differed from these public health and social agendas. In the meetings I observed, most members would not disclose or even discuss their experiences living with HIV. A number of women told me that if God wants their status to be known, he would make it happen. Muslims, they said, should not expose the secrets that God protects. I spoke to one woman about her reluctance to talk openly about her illness: if only God has the right to tell people you have this disease, why join an HIV support group in which you are obligated to disclose your status? She replied, "Even in the support group, you do not come out and say you have this disease. You only do so when you have a job to do."

I followed up, "What kind of job?" She said:

> Like the type of work we are doing with you. We are helping you because this will help you achieve your aims in school . . . even though we know you will not pay us. With others, no matter how much money they pay us, we will not disclose. It is only because we are used to you – that is the reason we do this. Since this group was first established, we do not usually tell people, even when we go out as a group to work. There are other groups that do that. They will be showing themselves and begging for alms. . . . You see some groups have governors or politicians that will give women clothes during *sallah* festival, but they never give us these things.[4]

In these women's support groups, business matters, rather than health concerns, dominated their discussions each month. The male leaders presided over the meetings, while many of the women listened quietly. Most would not participate. In individual interviews with these women, they told me that they disliked the politics and corruption that enveloped the support group's business and outreach efforts. Women implied and sometimes explicitly stated that they felt neither empowered nor encouraged by these programs. They had little interest in disclosing their status to one another, much less to public audiences.

"Why then would you continue to go?" I asked repeatedly.

Asabe, an HIV-positive widow in the group, then stated matter-of-factly that she joined the support group to find an HIV-positive husband:

> Now, I am well and healthy. I think I can live positively if I find someone with the same status. So, that is why I think of marriage. . . . My sister-in-law also says, "[Asabe], you are better now. You should get married. You are always covering yourself and making a hard, unfriendly face. How can any man be brave enough to approach you?" Any man who wants to marry me would have to talk to my family or close friends. In my mind, I know what my problem is, so I do not tell my sister-in-law anything.

I just laugh. I said to her, "Covering myself will not stop me from getting a husband." It has only been in the past months that I have thought about marriage and childbirth . . . I just pray for God to give me a responsible husband.

For women infected with HIV, marriage – and remarriage – is complicated. Northern men often accuse older single, "independent" women of promiscuity or even discredit them as lesbians. In Kano, they are sometimes derisively called *karuwai*, the Hausa term for prostitutes. And, because Nigerians frequently associate HIV with prostitution, women not only risk being marginalized because they have no husbands, but they also fear that these same people will suspect them of having the virus even when they show no symptoms. For these reasons, in addition to the cultural, religious, and economic importance of family, (re)marriage remains critical.

Women's understandable reluctance to disclose their status, however, presents a number of problems as they search for partners. Like Asabe's sister, family members, and friends unaware of their diagnosis will ask them questions about their boyfriends and arrange introductions to available men. Because they fear rejection, many women are unsure how to proceed in these potential relationships. Furthermore, even when they tell others about their virus, there are few people upon whom they can rely to help them find partners. Most Nigerians, I observed, would claim that they do not personally know an HIV-positive person, although they have their suspicions. HIV is far better understood as a symbol of social and moral crisis than it is a condition that affects ordinary people attempting to lead ordinary lives.[5]

Nevertheless, nonmarried women, like Asabe, hope that marriage will allay people's suspicions about both their character and HIV status, as well as their own personal anxieties about the future. Because disclosure is not necessary, many women see support groups as promising venues to meet men. HIV-positive women are less concerned with producing a "self-sufficient society" than they are with finding lasting, supportive relationships. The hopeful vision statements of support groups and the donors that fund them, in other words, do not necessarily align with those of women themselves. In what follows, I document a conversation I had in 2004 with women about their marriage plans.

"POSITIVE VOICES" SUPPORT GROUP

When I first met with the Positive Voices support group,[6] I learned that the stories women tell each other about the successful marriages of group members reaffirmed their beliefs that they too will find husbands. One example to which women continually referred was the marriage between Lantana and her husband, a former president of the support group. Soon after her first husband divorced her, and she received her diagnosis, Lantana's physician introduced her to her next husband. She told me:

> Time was not wasted. After two months of courting me, my husband's family sent his family to visit mine. They accepted. The marriage was tied [finalized] a week later. My life with him was beautiful. We had food: meat, chicken, milk . . . anything I wanted, he would provide it for me. I even misbehaved sometimes! You see he was old enough to be my father. My husband's friends would joke about how much he loved me. It was all he could talk about. I would never complain about him.

Lantana added that she was able to disclose her status to both her family and her community because of the security her marital status offered. Most women in this group desired a relationship trajectory similar to Lantana's marriage – where they no longer would be responsible for managing their day-to-day needs, and their fears of stigma would diminish as a result of their husbands' symbolic protection.

Other women would tell me that the HIV-positive men they met in their support groups were simply unacceptable. It was not uncommon for these men to take advantage of women's desperation for husbands. In addition, female members greatly outnumbered the male members in support groups. This imbalance provided lascivious men ample opportunities to have sex without committing to marriage. They would also often court multiple members of the group at the same time. Furthermore, because men and women alike sought to keep their sexual affairs secret, their actions were largely unsanctioned by their groups – even though everyone knew about them.

Over my 2004 visit, there was one particular HIV-positive man who was especially notorious for maltreating his support group girlfriends and wives. He had been previously engaged to another woman in the group

before being introduced to Habiba. He then broke off his engagement and
married Habiba instead. She described her marriage to this "womanizer":

> We met at a meeting. He said he loved me and wanted to know my
> house. . . . Although my father wanted me to wait a little longer, he later sent
> his parents and my dad agreed. . . . The only reason he gave for rushing to
> get married was to protect him from committing sin. That was why we got
> married so fast. I became pregnant after two months. I thought, I have got-
> ten this support group, I have a husband, and now I am pregnant, wow . . .
> [but] three months later we had problems and by five months the marriage
> was over. His problem was that if anything got between us, he would beat
> me. One day he came back home and I brought him food. No sooner had I
> turned to go get him a spoon, then he hit me with the lid of the plate on my
> head. He followed up with a beating. I just kept begging him for God's sake
> and the Prophet's sake, but he continued. . . . Afterwards, he handed me my
> divorce papers. . . . In my understanding there is nothing I can do.

During the time of this research, Habiba was seven months pregnant.
She had yet to go to an antenatal clinic to monitor her health or to receive
advice on to how to prevent transmitting HIV to her baby. Her former
husband has since moved on to a relationship with another woman and
expects to marry her.

Given the problems women like Habiba have in relationships with
HIV-positive men, they face a difficult dilemma over whether they can
have a boyfriend whose status is unknown to them. Their doctors and
counselors often echo these concerns over sero-discordant sexual partnerships – that is, those between HIV-positive and HIV-negative people. If
a woman marries an HIV-negative man and they do not use condoms, he
may contract the virus from her. Although antiretroviral therapies nearly
eliminate the possibility that an otherwise healthy HIV-positive woman
could pass on the virus, people still express a great deal of uncertainty over
the matter. Many northern Nigerian men, both Christian and Muslim,
refuse to use condoms. HIV-positive women cannot easily demand this
protection even when they fear exposing their partners to the disease.

And yet, because these women are commonly young, healthy, and indeed beautiful, men perpetually approach them and propose marriage.
In our group discussion one week, Hauwa summarized, "Everyday I get
someone interested in me. So long as I go out, then I will definitely get

someone professing his interest." These encounters often result in a string of excuses or lies. Another member of the group, Ladi, elaborated, "We positive women experience the problem of men wanting to marry us, wanting to have sex with us, but we do not tell them our status. I have many suitors. I tell them that my husband traveled to Saudi Arabia, so according to Islam, I have to wait for four years. If he does not return, then I can marry again."

A third woman, Hannatu, added:

> I know that since I am single, there will be times when I think about men. On those days, I get upset. But then, I find that even getting upset is useless. I cannot do anything about it. So I have solved the problem for myself by having sex with one of my HIV-positive boyfriends that I trust. I do not want to have sex with my negative boyfriend . . . I cannot marry the positive boyfriend because he has certain attitudes that do not fit into marriage . . . he is a womanizer. I can tolerate him from time to time just to satisfy my needs. I am only with him for that . . . definitely, I can be in love without having sex. In fact, I am in love with someone, but I wish to protect him.

In an interview with Asama'u later that month, she told me that she was in a relationship with an HIV-negative man and wanted to marry him but was unsure how to proceed:

> [My boyfriend] loves me like he could swallow me – so much so that he fights on my behalf! I made him take an HIV test, hoping he might turn out positive, but he was negative. I would tell him stories about marriages between positive and negative individuals just to test his frame of mind. He would say that even he could marry a positive person. I am afraid of telling him my status because I fear he will expose me to the community. . . . I sometimes think that I will marry him. Then, on our first night, I will tell him my status. I will request that he take another wife until I become cured. And then, we would live happily ever after. But, please understand that I have 30 different thoughts everyday over what to do about him. . . . Someone who does this for you [remaining married after learning his wife's HIV status] has done everything in the world for you! Even if he humiliates you, it is nothing. . . . After marriage, my precaution would be to use two condoms for every act so I can fully protect him. Because two condoms would mean that I am protecting the protection, since the outer condom might burst.

Asama'u married this boyfriend, and she gave birth to their first child in 2007. I never learned whether she ultimately disclosed her status. She was no longer active in the support group and only stayed in touch with other women when she collected her medications at the hospital. Her friends from the group told me that they were not sure of her husband's HIV status. Or, I thought, they might just have been unwilling to share it with me. I was also complicit in this secret, withholding the fact that I learned about his negative HIV result and her marriage dilemma a number of years ago.

As symptoms of HIV are not visible on their bodies, it is hard for non-married women to hide from men's attention, even if they wanted to do so. Men routinely flirt with them in schools, at their places of work, at parties, and at other events. The HIV-positive women I interviewed would quickly brush aside their advances when they found the men unattractive or undesirable. Still, these signs of affection pleased them. Once their boy-friends showed their intention to propose marriage, women found them-selves in a difficult position. Like Asama'u, they must discern whether their boyfriends' proposals are sincere and if they truly love these men in return. More critically, they wanted to know whether men would continue to support them and follow through with their marriage plans if they know they have the virus. These HIV-positive women's accounts of their relationship desires and experiences collectively reveal their willingness to assume great social and health-related risks in order to marry and have families.

As an anthropologist who has returned to northern Nigeria for short visits and extended months-long stays more than a dozen times in the past decade, I am continually reminded of both the constraints and privileges of following HIV-positive women's marriage pursuits. Often, I only met with them a few times over a brief period. I never learned whether or how they managed to resolve the conflicts they described to me with such rich detail. When I visited with Patience, the HIV counselor who introduced me to many of these women, I would ask whether she heard from them. Occasionally, I learned of their deaths. For example, Jummai and Mairo from Chapter Two passed away not long after I first interviewed them. Most, however, were alive, healthy, and so caught up in the everyday strug-gles of living their lives that they had little time for my visits.

There are a few women with whom I visit every time I travel to Nigeria. I know their homes and families as well as I know anyone in the country. Mostly, we chat lightheartedly, as close friends do: about our friends, work and school, movies, and politics. Our conversations gravitate to their love lives – as a result of the rapport we established over the years and the prominence of families in our shared hopes for the future. Because many of their friends and relatives still know little or nothing about their status, I do not take these intimate discussions for granted. I am aware of how difficult even these ordinary exchanges may be for them to have with others.

Women's descriptions, not only of their individual lives but also of the social worlds around them and how they have changed, helped me fill in gaps in my own understanding and provided nuance to my interpretations of other women's lives. Most importantly, I am drawn to their convictions: that they are trying to do the right thing and firmly believe that their diagnosis will not determine how they live their lives.[7] In the final two sections here, I focus on the stories of two of my close friends, Jamila and Elizabeth, who I have known since I first began this project.

JAMILA

"Tell me about your family and growing up," I began our interview. Jamila answered:

My father and my mother are from Sokoto State. He provided abundantly for us. My father brought our mother to Kano. She is Fulani and tall, while I am dark and take after my granny. Well, I used to be light-skinned, but I gradually darkened. There are nine of us children and I am the youngest among the females . . . I started secondary school, but I did not finish because I got married. At the time of the wedding, our dad had recently died. Otherwise, because I am the youngest, he would have let me continue with school. It was my mother's decision to have me married off. . . . Before my husband, I had a boyfriend who wanted to marry me, but it was not meant to be. He had even taken money to my parents. This man used to sell provisions (household goods) close to our house. He would send me on errands, and he started giving me gifts. Later, this man came to visit me. I would sit and chat with him until he sent me money to show his intentions. We were together until I got into Form Two. That is when I met the man I would eventually marry. I then stopped talking to him. . . . My husband also lived in the same area as me. One day, as I was passing by him with my friends from school, he saw me and introduced himself. From then on, he would greet me after school. He asked me where our house was and he started visiting me there. We then started talking about marriage. . . . When I turned sixteen, I knew I was in love with him. Between me and my God, nothing could separate us.

In Jamila's description of her childhood earlier in our conversation, she told me about how she was a very troublesome young girl who would fight with anyone who challenged her. I asked her then, "Did you change after you met this man?" Jamila said, "Oh yes!"

> I became cultured and calm. I stopped all the fighting and even stopped visiting my friends. When he came to see me, I would greet him and bring him water. I dressed very neatly. I used to let my feet get dirty, but then I began to scrub them thoroughly. I would finish also my chores long before he came. My sisters and I were taught how to cook and I wanted to perfect it. So, I was always in the kitchen. . . . My wedding was not too elaborate. There was dancing and celebrating, but not for long. Then, I was taken to my husband's house on a Sunday, preceding the wedding *fatiha*.

I pressed her to tell me more about the first time she had sex with her husband:

> When I was taken?! Okay . . . well, when I was taken, I did not know how it was going to happen. So, when he touched me and started to make love to me, I felt the pain. I screamed and kept asking him to get off me. Afterwards, when he got up to go to the bath, I ran out of the house to my aunt's place without even putting on a veil. From there, I was taken to my senior brother's house in the morning. His wife, of course, scolded me. I told her, "If I knew that this is how marriage would be, I would not have married!" She got me hot water to massage myself because I was really swollen. My brother also reprimanded me. His wife told me to use a jelly. They told my husband to be gentle. My aunt promised things would fit in a few days, to which I told her, "It will never fit!" From then on, I became a person who dreaded the nightfall, as I would say.

We then turned to a discussion about the time when she first began to fall sick:

> My stomach was swollen at the time, and people thought I was pregnant. When I ate meat and drank *fura* [a yogurt-like beverage], I felt better. Still, it took a long time for me to grow fatter. I would start to gain weight; then, I would wake up one morning and discover my body looked like I had just been drained [of my body mass]. Actually then, I used to go to bed with a plate of food next to me. In fact, there was a day that a rat got to my food

before I woke up! I was so frustrated and started to cry. . . . My husband
registered my name at the hospital just before he died. After his death, I
started to take the medications. That is how I learned about the support
group. I asked a staff member when they met. So, she said on Friday, but
I did not get to go until the next week. At the time, I had not completed
my *takaba* [60 or more days of mourning]. When I got there, I saw my
"relatives" – my brothers and sisters – and I was like, "What?!" Of course,
I had seen other patients at the hospital, but it was in this context that I
gradually started to look and feel better. Patience said to me that she had
thought I was an old woman at our first meeting, not knowing I was very
young. I now discovered that I still had a life, as opposed to the saying
that HIV is a "nearby grave."

In our next interview a few weeks later, Jamila and I discussed how her
support group arranges marriages among its members:

At our meetings, if a guy sees a woman and likes her, then he will talk to
her. Quite a number of us have gotten married and some are still together
now. The guy might speak to her directly or tell her friend. She would
then tell the person what she thinks. If she finds him okay, fine. But, if she
already has somebody outside of the group, then you, as her friend, will inform him. You will offer to introduce him to another woman, if he wants.
So that is what happens. Then, there are some men who are not after
marriage. You will see the signs of love and then no marriage! Especially if
they never truly loved their girlfriends. . . . Of course, there is competition
in getting husbands. If you get one, another woman will say, "May God
give me a husband too." When choosing a husband, you need to check for
religion or faith, language or tribe, and attitude. And, if they come as a
package, then good!

Jamila and I then discussed stigma. I wanted to know whether she also
thought about remarrying, given the discrimination women sometimes
face when people learn they are infected.

If people get to know my status, I will experience stigma. For example, if
we meet at ceremonies, people might not want to eat from the same tray
with me, or people will not want to handle something I touch. Or even sit
near me. They might leave when I sit next to them . . . so, at ceremonies
I would just get my own plate and move aside to eat alone, just to avoid
these scenarios. At home, I separated my things from other people's and
even my sleeping space. . . . I worry that no one will marry me. If people
run away from me, then who will desire me, much less have children with

me? I was just waiting for my death . . . but later, I improved and became healthier. I no longer worry so much and I am even contemplating marriage. I never thought I would get married until I joined the group. I was only concerned about my health. But when I saw that people were marrying, I became more comfortable with the idea. . . . I think about suitors every day. My parents or relatives bring up the issue of suitors like twice a week and marriage like three times in a week. I even get like two or three offers of marriage in a week. . . . Honestly, I do not think about having kids because I worry about the baby getting HIV at birth. My relatives only talk to me about marriage, not having kids, but they would love to see me have them.

Finally, I asked Jamila about whether she currently had any boyfriends.

My boyfriends right now? Even yesterday, a man followed me home. Now, I have two admirers. I told the man from yesterday that I would show him our house. But, in reality, I will not go out with him because he does not know my problem. The second suitor is also not really my type. He is on the big side and his language is also a barrier. No, I am not tribalist, you know. Before, I said that Hausas marry other tribes, but other tribes do not . . . I have had boyfriends of other tribes. It is just that, well, he is not the one for me. He discussed marriage, but I naturally do not like big men. I prefer medium-sized ones. A while back, there was another guy I met at the hospital, but he also did not fit my criteria. . . . To get a husband, I just need to maintain my dignity and respectability. Even outsiders can vouch for my character. I do not allow a man to know me as a woman [have sex]. I am neat and dress well.

When I visited Jamila nearly ten years later in 2014, we reminisced about how long we had known each other. I had returned to Kano in 2006, two years after our first meeting. A local nongovernmental organization had just hired Jamila to carry out home-based care in the same hospital where I conducted interviews. She rushed into and out of the clinic, collecting patients' names and visiting them in their houses. I learned that, around the time of our first interview, she met a man in the support group. Looking back on her relationship with this husband, Jamila recalled that he was not like the other men. Patience, who often went to visit her with me, agreed. He was one of the good ones.

Jamila's new boyfriend repaired computers for a living. He worked in the support group's offices. She fell in love and they married quickly. Within two months, Jamila was pregnant with her son. Although she had

two children previously with her first husband, his family took custody of
them upon his death and she no longer saw them. The second marriage,
she said, changed her life. He was a devoted, faithful husband who provided her the support she needed to meet her responsibilities as a wife.

Jamila threw herself into taking care of her husband. They both eagerly
anticipated the birth of their child. She seemed to know about the risk of
transmitting HIV to her baby; however, she said, she delivered her son at
home. Although Jamila enrolled in the hospital's HIV clinic, neither she
nor her baby took antiretroviral (ARV) therapies at the time of her delivery.
She did not offer me a reason why. I suspected she was on a waiting list, as
many women were at the time. Because she did not go to the hospital to
give birth, she did not receive the medications that are provided freely to
prevent mother-to-child transmission.

About the same time Jamila had her baby, her husband fell seriously
ill. He died just a couple months after the birth. Jamila returned to her
family's home with her son, deeply depressed. She felt hopeless, she told
me, after losing both of the men in her life. Her parents counseled her and
tried to make her feel better. They told Jamila that she was still healthy
and beautiful. She could marry again. Jamila then began to collect antiretroviral therapies through the clinic's treatment program. The hospital staff
tested her son for HIV when he turned six months, and he showed signs
of the virus's antibodies. This result suggested that he too was infected. It
was too early to confirm his status, but Jamila was devastated.

When I came back a year or so later, I learned that Jamila had left her
job and moved. I thought it was the last time I would hear from her. In
2010, however, Patience told me about Jamila's third husband. They had
married in 2009. One of the HIV-positive men who collected medications
in the hospital approached a counselor and asked for help finding a wife.
He noticed Jamila in the clinic and thought she was attractive. He pressed
for more details about her and the counselor introduced them.

Abdul was a young, handsome, and wealthy Hausa man who lived a
few hours' drive from the city of Kano. He was also the son of a *Tsarki*
(emir), the political and religious leader of the area. His title was *Hakimi*,
or a traditional district head. Abdul and Jamila exchanged phone numbers
and they spoke frequently. He asked her if he could visit her at her house
and she agreed. Then, they quickly fixed a date for the wedding. When
Jamila saw his house for the first time, its beauty and size surprised her.

She did not know he came from such a privileged background. No one in his family knew his status, and she carefully protected his secret. Abdul divorced his first wife because, after seven years of marriage, she could not give him children. When Jamila first became pregnant, the whole family celebrated. Abdul was also relieved because it proved he was not infertile.

When I heard that Jamila had given birth, I asked Patience if we could go and visit her. Jamila and Abdul enthusiastically told us to come. When we arrived in the city, Abdul picked us up at the bus stop in his Mercedes. He wore sunglasses and a *baban riga* (traditional Hausa attire). We drove into a residential area and pulled up in front of a richly adorned house, painted light green. Patience and I entered into the courtyard, and they ushered us into the parlor. The house's generator powered a satellite television and an electric fan in a small but lavishly decorated parlor. Jamila came into the room with her daughter and son to greet us. She glowed. Jamila wore a light green dress – her favorite color, I recalled. Her daughter was eighteen months old, and the son from her second marriage was around four.

Jamila tearfully told us that the laboratory repeated her son's HIV screening at eighteen months, and he tested negative. After their marriage, Abdul adopted him and treated him exactly the same as he would his own son. He paid for his school fees, health care, and clothes and showed him genuine kindness and pride. Only the neighbors and friends who knew Abdul before their marriage were aware that he was not his biological child. That day, we ate the food she prepared and played with the baby. We exchanged gifts and took photos. Jamila clearly thrived in her new home.

In 2014, Patience and I returned once again to visit them. Over the four years that passed, Abdul and Jamila gave birth to a second baby girl, who was then nearly two years old. Jamila not only returned to school and completed her secondary school certificate, but she advanced beyond that and recently received a postsecondary school diploma. Her husband helped her find a job as a civil servant in the Ministry of Education.

I told her that I wanted to use the story of her marriage at the end of my book, because I thought it was important that people read about HIV-positive women who found love again. She agreed and helped me fill in some of the details about her life that I had not known. Jamila emphasized that when she first married Abdul, she never imagined that marriage could give her such joy. She assumed that she would suffer just as she had in her previous relationships. But, Abdul loves her so much, she said, and he loves her children. He paid for her education and assisted her in securing a job. She was truly happy, she repeated to me. Jamila hopes to have more children and work to improve schools across northern Nigeria.

I asked Jamila if there was anything she wanted to add. She said she would like to offer her advice to other HIV-positive women who were told that there is no hope for them. Initially, that was how she felt, not realizing, in fact, that her future would be so bright. When she let herself feel hopeful again, her whole story changed, she told me. Jamila wants women to know that their futures can also be bright. They should just keep their faith.

ELIZABETH

In 2003, I carried out an interview with Elizabeth, who I befriended in a support group in Jos. I began by asking her to tell me more about herself and her boyfriends growing up.

> I am from Plateau State of Nigeria and I am Berom by tribe . . . I am single now, but I hope to get married someday. I was thirteen when I started having boyfriends. I would just meet up with them and occasionally we would have sex. In 1992, when I was sixteen, I had a fight with my mom over one of these boyfriends – that I was too young and I should just focus on my studies. Of course, I was able to stay away from them for a while. But, when I got to SS2 [my second year of secondary school], I started again. You know the anxiety of adolescence. You want to feel like you belong.

After discussing her teenage years at length, she said she soon met the boyfriend who infected her with HIV. "How did you learn this?" I asked.

> Well, I got to know that I was infected in 2000. I had a boyfriend, who I started dating in 1994. I thought he was very serious about me, so I decided to stop my relationships with other boyfriends and stick to him. . . . Things were moving along fine. He even said he would marry me. I think that was in 1997. So, I just saw myself as his wife. I did not know that he was also seeing many other girlfriends then.

Elizabeth continued:

> Then, I introduced him to my family. We traveled together to his village and visited his grandparents. I was just like his wife. His sisters even called me, "our wife." Everybody thought he was going to marry me. And everything

was okay until 2000. Then, I fell severely ill. I lost weight – almost 10 kilograms. I went to the hospital and was treated for malaria. After that, I got better. Then, I started coughing. My mom said that I should go for a TB test. I said no, but she insisted.... So, I got dressed and we went to the hospital. The doctor asked me some questions. He said that I should go for an HIV test. I said there is no need because I only have sex with my boyfriend. I do not sleep around. But I just said to myself, "Let me just do it and learn my HIV status anyway."

My boyfriend came back and I told him that I went for an HIV test.... He said, if it turns out positive, he would kill me and kill himself. I was very sure that it was not going to be positive. So, I went to collect the result. The doctor said that there is a problem. The test is reading reactive. I said, "What is that? What is the meaning of reactive?" He said that I should go for a confirmation test. I became very anxious. I went home, picked up money, and took a taxi to Plateau Hospital for the Western blot test.

Luckily, I knew the person there who gave these tests. He took a blood sample and told me to come back after three days. I told my boyfriend about it. He said that I should not collect the test result. I told him that I needed to see it, so I could know what my problem is and how to face it. Of course, I cried and cried and prayed and fasted. I said to God that I would try to use my life better, if he gives me this chance. I then thought I would just kill myself if positive, because I cannot watch myself die like that . . . because of the way AIDS dehumanizes you at the mercy of other people. You are just helpless.

On the day I collected the result, I heard the guy just talking, talking. I knew then that it was positive. Somehow, the few days of waiting gave me a little courage.... So, he started telling me things about HIV and how I can respond to it positively. I cried and I took the result to my doctor. He told me that the drugs are very expensive.

I was supposed to attend a fellowship at church that day, so I went. I was not myself and everybody noticed. After the fellowship, the president asked what was wrong with me. I said that I was okay. My boyfriend too was in the fellowship. He saw me, and he knew it was positive. So, he asked, "Is it true?" and I said, "Yes, it is positive, so you better go and get your test and learn what to do with your life. As for me, I am positive. Go and do your own." He tried to assure me that there was no problem. Even if he started dating me before this problem, he said, this would not scare him away. I said again, "Go and do your test." He told me no and started giving me excuses . . . I had to drag him to the hospital. He was also positive.

Elizabeth then described to me how she began to tell others and find help and support:

I told my brother-in-law because I was staying with them. I was very close with him . . . I continued to lose weight and people kept asking me, "What is wrong with you?" You know Nigerians become very suspicious. . . . So, there was this time I had pneumonia and it was very bad. I did a test for malaria and I had the parasite. I treated it, but then later in the evening I started vomiting blood. I said, "Today, my own (life) has finished." I thought I was going to die. I told my neighbor, who was a nurse. She said that I should go to the hospital. This is not just malaria. I then went to the casualty unit.

The next day, I was okay . . . I had a TB test, but it was negative . . . so I decided to stop going about like that – ignoring my symptoms and not telling anyone I was infected. One day, I just discussed it with my friend, who was also a doctor. I told him that I hoped to save money for antiretrovirals. . . . He said he was going to talk it over with someone. Whatever the outcome, he would let me know. He discussed it with another doctor and he said he was going to help me. I brought him my test results and he gave me medications. I started recovering and gaining weight.

Then, last year, this doctor told us patients that we are going to form a support group. People (with this sickness) are getting to be too many and he cannot keep up. He felt it was better to have a group where we can just get together and discuss our problems . . . so we started meeting every Sunday. Sometimes, we are invited to go out and give testimonies. Our intention is to reach students and tell them that this disease is real. There are many people out there who are just dying in silence. We told them, "Do not die in silence. Come let us do something that will improve our lives. This is not the end of life. HIV is just a disease. There are so many people who die every day, who do not have HIV. The virus is not a death sentence." . . . Of course, I do not have to tell people that I am positive. If you start to tell everybody, you will feel hurt and it will stress you out. I talk about the disease a lot, but I do not have to say I am positive.

Although I think Elizabeth wanted to end her interview there, I wanted to know more about her boyfriend. "Were you still with him? What happened?" I asked.

After he found out that he was positive, he did not actually kill himself, nor did he try to kill me. I talked to him. I said that we can still live positively. . . . Later, I discovered that he was not faithful to me. So I called him and confronted him. I told him that this is what I heard, and I wanted him to tell me the truth about it. He fed me lies, saying that it was not true. I said to him, "We have come a long way. There is nothing I cannot do." I would have forgiven him, if he told me the truth. I would have known he accepted that it was his fault and he was willing to change. But, he was not willing. I told him we should call off the relationship.

When we concluded the interview that day, Elizabeth told me a final story:

There was a day I was walking down the street, and I met a guy. He said he wanted to know my house. I refused to show him, but he insisted. So I said I would just meet him somewhere. I was with my medications that day. I then showed him the drugs, and I told him straight out that I am HIV positive. He still did not believe me. He said I should follow him to a hotel. And I told him, "No!" I was afraid, though, so we went to one restaurant. We sat there and chatted. He said that if I had followed him to the hotel, he would have forced me to sleep with him. Men think you say that you have HIV to scare them away. . . . Some people that have it, they choose to be wicked and just spread it all around. You will not know who is positive. But I cannot be that wicked. They say, "Somebody gave it to me, so I am going to spread it too." So, thousands do that. But if they know that they can live positively with the virus, it would reduce their evil thoughts about it. They would just live their normal life. . . . I want HIV-positive people to be more optimistic about life. Before there was no cure for pneumonia or even malaria, but now there are ways out. People should just have hope. Who knows whether something will just come up? By the grace of God, you will see that it is over. One day, you will see that we have made it. I have hope that one day there will be treatment for us.

With the exception of a few years between 2002 and 2014, I visited Jos annually and I met with Elizabeth each time. Over the first few years, she continued to advance in her degree program in hotel and restaurant management. Soon, she moved out of her family's house into a small apartment with a kitchen. Elizabeth could then formally begin her own business. She found financial support for her bakery from a series of generous boyfriends. One of the kindest of these boyfriends was an older, married man. He would help her whenever she asked. Elizabeth said she knew that condoms could protect her partners and she insisted on using them.

Another man – an Igbo from Anambra State – fell in love with her, Elizabeth described. As their relationship progressed, she disclosed her status to him. Although he was surprised, he wanted to stay with her. We joked over Igbo men's reputations for their intense emotions. They fought constantly. Eventually, she ended the relationship, but he continued to pursue her. He would bring up her HIV status every time he tried to reconcile with her. I was unsure, from Elizabeth's description, whether he did this in an attempt to display his trustworthiness or if it served as a threat – that he could use this information to discredit her, if he wanted. Either way, it made her acutely uncomfortable.

While the support group served as such a valuable resource for her in 2003, things began to change. As the number of patients grew, the meetings' intimate dynamics that led to so many friendships in its early years gave way to large, impersonal lectures. In addition to becoming the first treatment center in Nigeria to be awarded PEPFAR funding in 2004, the clinic garnered the support of large American churches, which routinely sent volunteers to the hospital. Initially, some of the support group members built relationships directly with donors. If they had a particular need, one of these patrons might give them money. However, the hospital's policy stipulated that all donations must first go to the administrators. Allegations of corruption abounded. Elizabeth once asked the group for help with her school fees and she was turned down. Then, she began to question what she gained through her participation. Slowly, she withdrew from the group. Elizabeth now goes to the clinic only when she needs to collect her medications.

In November 2013, I returned to Jos and arranged to have lunch with Elizabeth. Nearly two years had passed since our last visit and I was eager to hear her news. I invited another friend to come with me and we drove to the intersection where she said someone would wait to meet us. As we turned the corner, a young man noticed us immediately and waved. He introduced himself as David, and he entered the car to direct us to their house. I saw Elizabeth waiting for us at the gate. She wore an oversized polo shirt, and I commented to my friend that she had gained some weight. I went to greet her and it became clear that Elizabeth had not simply added weight: she was pregnant. We squealed and embraced each other. Although they had not formally wed yet, she said David was her husband, and he was indeed the father.

I wanted to know more about him but could not say much while he was in front of us. David was as intelligent and quick-witted as Elizabeth. Their chemistry was palpable. He was married once before, she later told me. His wife was unfaithful to him. When he approached his church to dissolve the marriage, David told her, they denied his request. He left her and the organization where he worked and moved to Jos, where he sought employment as a mechanical engineer. In his spare time, he was an amateur inventor. When David served in Nigeria's Youth Service Corps, a require-ment for university graduates, he received an award for creating a device used to purify water. When we met that week, he was working on another device to detect car theft.

As we spoke that afternoon, I looked for signs that might indicate whether Elizabeth had disclosed her status to David. There was one point in the conversation that gave me pause. I had just recovered from a bad case of malaria and we were discussing how to prevent the illness. Elizabeth told me that, unlike her, David gets malaria all the time. He admired the fact that she takes such good care of him when he falls ill. He said that she would wake him up when he falls asleep on the couch to make sure he slept under the mosquito net in their bedroom. Although they did not mention HIV then, David and Elizabeth's concern for one another's well-being show-cased the aspirations that all HIV-positive women express as they consider the consequences of disclosing their status to partners. I felt fairly confident then that the two of them shared this intimate knowledge with one another.

I went back to Jos again in March 2014 to stay with Elizabeth for a few days. When I arrived, she was rushing to complete a cake for one of her customers. Although Elizabeth looked as if she might give birth at any point, they still had nearly a month left to wait. David did not have full-time employment, so the couple relied primarily on her income to support them. "When you run your own business," she said, "there are no maternity leaves."

This visit, we had a chance to speak alone. I asked Elizabeth to tell me everything about David: "How did you meet? What is his story?" She said her neighbor introduced them. He had just arrived in Jos and collected her mobile number. They were casual friends for about a year, talking on the phone and occasionally meeting up for a drink. David then confessed to Elizabeth that he was in love with her and wanted to get married. When she sensed he was serious, she knew she had to tell him her status. He was taken aback by her disclosure but had no intention of leaving her. Together, they went for a test. David received a negative result. Elizabeth's viral load was undetectable. She had been on continuous treatment for over a decade, carefully adhered to her medication regimen, and was otherwise healthy. She also knew that it was more difficult for a woman to pass HIV to a man than for a man to give the virus to a woman.

Nevertheless, they found it difficult to use condoms consistently. David disliked them, Elizabeth explained. He described the experience as akin to "eating candy with the wrapper still on it." Furthermore, David wanted to have a baby and did not want Elizabeth to use contraception. She conceived less than a year after they started having sex. He was elated over the news of her pregnancy and doted on her. After going for a scan, they learned they were going to have a girl, although they did not entirely trust the lab technician. While at least three weeks remained, Elizabeth and David already had their bag for the hospital packed.

Elizabeth's concession that she could not force her husband to use condoms sat uncomfortably with me, given how committed I knew she was to them when she was younger.[8] Yet, in our conversation about her upcoming third-trimester appointment, she raised an important point. Then, she and her husband would go together to the hospital to be screened for HIV again. Elizabeth felt particularly happy that David would receive another test. He had not gone to the clinic since August, when they first found out she was pregnant. She thought that his excitement over fatherhood might motivate him to take better care of his own health, including being more open to condoms and family planning in the future.

We spoke in detail about their preparations. Although Elizabeth felt ready, she was nervous. A few months earlier, she had deep pains in her stomach and they thought she might have had premature contractions. When they did another scan, the doctors found a large cyst pressing up against her womb. This could complicate the delivery, Elizabeth said, particularly if she needed a Caesarian section. David and Elizabeth opted to give birth at the teaching hospital. Although the costs would be greater than other hospitals or clinics, they knew they would have access to a specialist if they needed it.

Another major hospital in Jos was conducting a clinical trial on the reproductive health outcomes of sero-discordant couples. David and Elizabeth qualified, but they were skeptical. In exchange for joining the trial, the doctors said they could give birth at the hospital for free. But, they had heard many stories of malpractice in this particular hospital. David and Elizabeth were also reluctant to enroll in the trial because they would have to regularly go to appointments, where they would be subjected to a number of tests. The benefits, Elizabeth thought, did not outweigh the risks. And finally, she had a business to run and did not have time for this additional stress.

While most of our conversations over those days centered on Elizabeth's pregnancy, we also talked about her progress with her work. That year, she finally opened her own shop. The bakery was located on a busy street about a twenty-five-minute walk from her house. Inside the shop, there was a large refrigerator displaying several cakes. Elizabeth had just hired a salesgirl. One of the benefits of having the bakery outside her house, she explained, was that she no longer relied on her friends and family as her primary customers. It allowed her to avoid awkward encounters with family members who refused to pay her for her services. Her new customers could see the sign above her shop and walk in to inquire about her baked goods. Elizabeth told me she hopes to travel to the United States one day for a course in a culinary school, where she would learn some of the professional techniques that she saw on the television show, *Cake Boss*.

In mid-April 2014, I received a call. Elizabeth gave birth to a girl. She and the baby were healthy, and they had returned home from the hospital. Despite his bouts of nervousness, David did not need to be hospitalized alongside her, Elizabeth jokingly confirmed to me. Both were thrilled to finally have their own family.

POSITIVE LIVING

HIV-positive women in northern Nigeria are staunchly committed to asserting their roles and responsibilities as wives and mothers. While the virus's inexorable stigma threatens to strip them of the virtue they secure through these social positions, Jamila and Elizabeth display remarkable resilience as they have lived with HIV for over thirteen years. The women in this chapter firmly believe that their plans for the future will not be thwarted by their positive diagnosis, despite their partners' betrayals, maltreatment, and subsequent deaths.

From the time they were first diagnosed to the present, Jamila and Elizabeth's hopefulness only grew. Their declarations shifted from the things they hoped were *no longer* on their horizon – an invisible death, rejection, and abandonment – to broader questions of what their lives might hold: "Who knows whether something will just come up?" Elizabeth asked in that first meeting. The possibilities they considered expanded with each of my subsequent visits: from vague statements about making improvements in their lives to intimate relationships and the chance of finding husbands. Marriage, in turn, allowed them to imagine the previously unthinkable prospect of healthy children. And finally, completing their education inspired them to dream about what they could accomplish through their work – a flourishing business and travel to the United States for advanced training in Elizabeth's case, and improving the lives of others in the state by reforming education in Jamila's account.

Jamila and Elizabeth fulfilled their goals of finding husbands, giving birth, finishing school, and obtaining meaningful and profitable work. Their husbands, in turn, have shown them affection, economic support, fidelity and generosity, and pride in their growing families. Each couple cared for one another's health, as well as their emotional and sensual needs, inspiring a sense of belonging, protection, and empowerment. Jamila and Elizabeth both emphasized that all women should keep their faith in God and not lose hope – a cure for HIV is on the horizon. In the meantime, they can live virtuous, normal lives and find happiness with loving families. To repeat Jamila's point: when she let herself feel hopeful again, her whole story changed.

Read together, Jamila and Elizabeth's relationship narratives offer an important illustration of the ways in which global health campaigns dedicated to funding HIV treatment and care in Nigeria intercede in these women's expectations for the future. Many HIV-positive people are now confident that their deaths are not foretold and a cure is forthcoming because of the level of health they have attained and maintained through their access to antiretroviral therapies. And yet, as evident above, the stories these women shared with me about what they want for their lives and the particular constraints they face diverged, at times, from the hopeful rationales that underscore these public health interventions.

Often implicitly understood in donor-funded projects is the idea that, if patients openly acknowledge their HIV status to others, they will challenge public misperceptions surrounding the virus and thus reduce their stigma. Their advocacy efforts might even produce lasting political change as leaders become more responsive to Nigerians' health care needs. Unquestionably, support groups and other associations of persons living with HIV/AIDS have been highly visible across the country, playing a key role in public campaigns for the rights of persons living with HIV. These campaigns have sought to counter popular misunderstandings and raise political awareness through interviews, testimonials, radio programs, dramas, rallies, and other projects.

Nevertheless, members of the groups I observed frequently felt that the risks of exposing themselves were too great and the threat of stigma from their families, friends, and neighbors might even increase. Many women ambivalently participated in support group initiatives because they provided them financial support. Very few of the women I met felt they could rely on these sources of income over the long term, however, nor did they want to depend on them.

Support group marriages, in contrast, provide one potentially effective way of countering the virus's stigma and gaining the interpersonal support they seek. Through the group's collective recognition of women as social and sexual beings – as opposed to polluted, diseased, and abandoned individuals – HIV-positive women were encouraged to pursue these larger life goals of reconstituting families. By attending support group meetings, even if not actually disclosing their status, women sought to locate men who would not reject them. Many of them found attentive and kindhearted partners through these groups. Not all of these relationships have happy endings, however. The same structural forces and experiences of intimate violence that first led to women's infection may continue to haunt them in subsequent marriages.

HIV-positive women also seek relationships with partners whose status may be unknown to them. These decisions reflect their conviction that they are, in fact, acting in good faith, as Elizabeth plainly sought to convey to me. Although we did not discuss it specifically, the World Health Organization's 2012 guidelines on counseling sero-discordant couples recommended precisely the actions that she and David took.[9] They received HIV counseling and testing that supported mutual disclosure. Although antiretroviral therapies do not eliminate the risk of transmission entirely, they do dramatically decrease the virus's infectiousness – so much so that these medications are heralded as both treatment and prevention. Elizabeth and David are not alone in this predicament over whether HIV-positive and HIV-negative couples can safely have sex. Epidemiologists suggest that, in sub-Saharan Africa, as many as half of all HIV-positive people in cohabiting relationships are in sero-discordant relationships.[10]

HIV-positive women who marry HIV-positive men hope to attain a safer, stable, and more predictable future – that is, one in which they do not have to disclose their status and thus risk rejection. Then, they cannot infect new partners, and they believe these relationships lower the chance that people will stigmatize them. Other HIV-positive women hope for partners who they genuinely love and are loved by in return, regardless of status – even if the medical and social risks are greater. They do not see their choices in men as reflections of inconsiderate, dangerous, or even immoral behavior, as others might judge them. Rather, they are committed to caring for their husbands and cultivating a better future for their families – as normal and healthy people do – with minimal fears over whether HIV will irreparably damage their lives. Their hopes are thus shaped by, and in turn engender, deeply social, intimate, and embodied meanings and experiences.

Conclusion: Evidence and Substance

There is substance in the gathering
of bodies battered by this disease.
There is evidence in the quiet promise
we make to be here again next week.
There is substance in the sweet taste
of coconut water, the scent of morning.
There is evidence in the songs a slim man
sings, healing as the balm of warmed oil.
There is substance in the expletives shattering
our peace, the tears, the lament, the fear.
There is evidence in the hum of recognition,
the comfort of hands held tightly.
There is substance in the streets walked
to tell people to hope for tomorrow.

Kwame Dawes, *Faith*

Throughout this book, I have documented the centrality of hope in HIV-positive women's narratives of their lives: for health and well-being; for love, marriage, and children; for education, work, and economic prosperity; and for security and longevity. Through an ethnographic lens, I have located these dreams in women's lived realities. Their aspirations for the future surface in scenes of youthful trysts and romantic encounters; in marriage celebrations and fearful wedding nights; in violent encounters with abusive husbands and futile pleas for help from family members; in hidden pregnancies and joyous presentations of baby pictures; in elaborate beauty regimens and conspicuous displays of generosity to relatives, neighbors, and researchers; in successful entrepreneurial businesses and uncompensated, arduous household labor. These women's steadfast faith – in God, in the virtue of family, in a meaningful life, in a cure for their disease – grounds these hopes as they face formidable daily struggles. Amid the changes ushered in by global initiatives centered on increasing access to HIV treatment and medical services in Nigeria, theirs is a story of continuity.

HIV-positive women's striking beauty and virtuous acts not only vividly highlight their respectability; they also complement the effects of antiretroviral therapies in concealing their disease. Regardless of the circumstances surrounding how they became infected, the virus's close association with promiscuity and immorality requires them to carefully monitor their reputations. These women, I have shown, protect their character by hiding their husbands' lack of support, violent dispositions, extramarital affairs, and poor health, among other traits and behaviors that might lead people to question the integrity of their marriage. They go to great lengths to protect their own and their partners' secrets – even when these silences, lies, and pretenses threaten to expose them to greater harm.

No singular case guided the narrative arc of this book, nor did I intend to suggest that the virus necessarily follows a predictable path as it becomes interwoven in a woman's life trajectory. Nevertheless, I observed patterned features in HIV-positive women's experiences, which informed the major themes of this text.

First, I found that the structural forces that reproduce social inequalities – specifically, the ability of men to exert their power and control over women – affect the strategies that youth employ as they navigate financial hardships and their desires for love, dignity, and respect. These acts involve the conspicuous presentation of some features of their relationships and discretion over others. For example, men may shower their girlfriends with gifts, including candies, cloth, jewelry, and other luxurious items, in addition to paying for their school fees and even changing their grades. In exchange, they seek intimacy, sex, and sometimes marriage. Young women, in turn, may accept their admirers' gifts but refuse to speak with them, in a display of timidity or shyness. Or, they may blatantly lie to maneuver around men's persistent attention. They conceal these relationships to escape the scrutiny of their parents and family members. They also hide the fact that they may have multiple boyfriends, each of whom meets different needs or desires. These same tactics that women employ to negotiate competing pressures surrounding love and sex before testing positive for HIV are also relied upon after contracting the virus, as we have seen.

Second, I suggested that marriage is a process rather than an event and described how such an understanding helps elucidate why HIV is transmitted between husbands and wives. Weddings, for instance, take place within a larger matrimonial economy, in which an array of material and symbolic resources are exchanged. Through marriage, men and women assume new identities, which entail a particular set of rights, responsibilities, and allocations of power. As these values, relationships, and institutions are socially reproduced, gender power inequalities are exacerbated. Wives take on increasing responsibility for attending to the needs and demands of their husbands, even when their children's and their own needs go unmet. And, when women lack the capacity to carry out this labor, they risk losing their husbands and children. Men may remarry, pronounce a divorce [talaka], or simply jettison their wives for other women.

Like women's early relationships, marriages are characterized by tensions between the things husbands and wives share with one another and the things they hide. Women may actively hide their partners' secrets – such as acts of infidelity, violence, infertility, neglect, and HIV transmission – even when men refuse to do the same for them. They defend these dominant and dominating masculine privileges in sometimes-futile efforts to salvage power, enact respectability, and secure their health and well-being.

Third, I illustrated the effects of HIV-positive diagnoses on women's family life. HIV-infected patients grapple with a set of difficult questions: What is the virtuous thing to do with this secret and deeply discrediting knowledge once it is in their possession? To whom, when, why, and how should they share information about their HIV status? In short, how do people uphold their dignity through speech? Some of the most common ways women attempt to carry out these social goals, I learned, are through the strategic use of silence, lies, and indirect communication. What goes unsaid is just as important as what is said. For instance, one of the women in the clinic pretended not to understand English in her coun-seling session to establish a position of plausible deniability. By denying knowledge of her status, she could potentially evade being held responsi-ble for spreading the virus. Women also use speech acts to perform gen-dered identities and to assume greater power within their relationships. Ultimately, they aim to display their virtue and present themselves as ethical persons.

Fourth, I highlighted the significance of women's bodies in their nar-ratives as they sought to meet embodied, emotional, and sensual needs of others. This labor is essential, women stressed, to securing not only their own well-being but also the welfare of their families. Their bodies serve as a means of production from which they generate both material and symbolic capital. One woman's eye-catching beauty, for instance, was a means of attracting the attention of potential customers. She would sell the clothes off her back to other women who also sought to enhance their appearance and desirability. Those who occupy these sales and service positions are implicitly or explicitly expected to offer their committed attention to clients, to flirt with or amuse their customers, or to exhibit intimate knowledge about others' bodies in order to generate an income. Even wives who lack employment in the formal economy are called upon to attend to the needs of their husbands and to provide hospitable envi-ronments for their families and guests. Domestic spaces serve as symbolic extensions of women's bodies. HIV-positive women hoped that these ef-forts would not only secure them support for their subsistence; they were also a means of financing their future aspirations – school fees, business investments, and health care expenses, among others.

Many women believe that HIV devalues their bodies, while the virus simultaneously produces a new set of demands upon them. They often give more of themselves – their money, time, and labor – than they intend to give out of fear of jeopardizing precarious relationships with their partners and families. And should their bodies betray them, women risk not only exposing their HIV status but also severing sources of income and social ties with others. These bodily and caregiving practices reveal how ethics become embedded in their exchanges with others.

And fifth, while HIV-positive women were indeed using both speech and their bodies to present themselves as ethical persons, I also showed how these efforts became enmeshed in larger goals of finding love and (re)constituting families. Marriage and reproduction serve multiple purposes; most critically, these social processes are the primary ways in which northern Nigerian women fulfill gendered and religious expectations, as well as cement their reputations as respectable persons. Husbands, HIV-positive women hope, will alleviate some of the burden of managing their day-to-day needs and expenses. Furthermore, because HIV still is popularly and erroneously believed to be a disease that is concentrated among single, promiscuous youth, few people suspect that a married woman could be infected with the virus. With the support of their husbands, HIV-positive women are often better able to protect themselves from their status being exposed without their consent.

Lastly, many women expect that if their families see they are able to marry a caring husband and have children despite being HIV-positive, they will no longer be stigmatized. They also think it would be easier to disclose their status as married women than as unmarried women. The final chapter presented life histories of two women who found husbands, had children, completed school, and located rewarding work – achieving the social goals that all Nigerian women desire for themselves and their daughters. Not only do HIV-positive women dream of these life trajectories, they actually attain them. Through families, women secure both their privacy and a sense of hope for the future.

What do these stories teach us, more generally, about the lives of women and families in sub-Saharan Africa? What can we learn from them that might contribute to advancing the aims of public health programs and improving the delivery of medical services to this population?

Across popular and philanthropic accounts of HIV-positive women in Africa, two tropes dominate. The first casts the "African woman" as a heroic figure in the face of patriarchy, disease, and widespread social inequalities. In the second account, she is a passive victim of both individual men and a larger system of patriarchy firmly rooted in a generic "African culture." By emphasizing women's powerless positions within their marriages, families, workplaces, and the state, these victim narratives invite global interventions to save them. Likewise, these counternarratives present women as strong, assertive, and independent protagonists, whose defiant acts parallel the experiences and achievements of Western feminists.

Anthropologists have critiqued these theoretical trajectories, arguing that the resistance/subordination binary does not capture the range of motivations, desires, and goals that women possess. Sexual partners, in particular, reveal critical ways through which women attempt to situate themselves in gendered political and moral orders. As fatal medical prognoses, stigmatizing public sentiments, and economic constraints collide to exclude HIV-positive people from the social category of virtuous personhood, northern Nigerian women imagine and produce new futures for themselves and their families.

This book thus challenges readers to consider how HIV-positive women endeavor to enact hope and dignity in their everyday lives. "Virtue" is not a static set of criteria to which people do or do not measure up. Rather, virtues are interwoven in an array of motivations, bodily practices, and the ordinary sensibilities that women apply as they attempt to figure out how to live respectable lives with a deeply stigmatizing disease. And, as they strive to carry out their plans, HIV-positive women work diligently upon their sense of self. They take care of their partners, families, and customers, using their bodies, speech, emotions, and hard-earned material resources. They forge new modes of survival and they seek out novel ways of producing intimacy within their relationships.

In many respects, women's responses to HIV are no different from their reactions to the other numerous social and physiological threats they encounter over the life course. However, the virus *does* disrupt women's lives in ways that make them vulnerable to a greater burden of suffering than that of HIV-negative individuals. Women suffer more than men, and poor women face more than wealthier ones. When couples learn their status, feelings of fear, anger, guilt, and shame lead to intense quarrels and marital dissolutions. As HIV-positive women move out of old relationships and into new ones, they have much to lose.

Reflecting a theme that has had a venerable history in West African scholarship – namely, secrecy and the associations between secrets and power – the HIV-positive women in this text have shown that secrets might actually be used as protection against oppression and exploitation. The act of safeguarding a partner's secret might in fact be seen as a

virtuous gesture; when these secrets are exposed, women may be disproportionately harmed. Secrets index both particular qualities of relationships – such as intimacy, trust, guilt, and fear – and the power relations
underscoring questions of who has the right to knowledge about others,
as well as how, when, and where this information can be revealed.

There are differences between Christianity and Islam regarding the ethical imperative of discretion, self-censorship, and public testimonials. The
Muslim women in my study, for example, widely believed that it is only God,
the all-knowing, who can expose secrets. Muslims must act with restraint
in both speech and bodily gestures so as not to reveal their own or others'
secrets in contexts they feel are deemed inappropriate by God. Christians,
in contrast, often see confession as a mechanism for transforming a person's life. Nevertheless, a number of women pointed out to me that these
statements should only be made in the context of an appropriate confessor,
who can share the burden of their secrets and help them find resolutions.
The complex relations between secrecy and revelation among northern
Nigerian women have important implications for public health programs.

How does this book's relatively small number of narratives help us
understand the larger global health and medical systems through which
HIV-positive women navigate? Too often in public health analyses of the
HIV pandemic, individual risk factors, choices, and behaviors are privileged over the ways in which these risks and experiences are determined
by social, economic, and political structures. Indeed, as anthropologists
have demonstrated, the spread of HIV over time is enmeshed in global
flows of capital, technologies, ideas, and people both into and out of Africa. As the International Monetary Fund and World Bank–led structural
adjustment programs have reconfigured regional economies across the
continent, state funding for medical infrastructure has declined precip-
itously, among other transformations in the provision of public goods
and services. In the wake of these changes, social and economic inequalities have proliferated. HIV risk maps onto these deep structural fissures.

The invisibility of HIV-infected patients in the early years of the epidemic in Nigeria was a product of global and state-level inaction, where
basic human rights were routinely withheld from the persons who needed
these protections the most. In the face of this neglect, HIV-positive patients, their partners, families, and activists have fought for political rec-

ognition, access to medical care, and pharmaceuticals. They aim to find spaces for hope and the means to escape a grim clinical, social, and political prognosis.

The women in this book provided insight into their relationships, instructive to public health professionals, counselors, and advocates in communities of persons living with HIV both within Nigeria and globally. Love and exchange, for example, are intertwined features of intimate relationships across Africa. Public health campaigns warn women about the risks of engaging in relationships with "sugar daddies." They suggest that these exchanges of gifts for sex with older men are inimical to the companionate – and *healthy* – relationships that they should enter. Religious and popular responses to these messages in Nigeria have taken this a step further: these relationships are not merely unsafe; they are also immoral.

And yet, it is important also to ask what these gifts symbolically mean, beyond their function or use value. If a man courts a woman without giving her something, it could suggest that he is not sincere in his desire to marry her. Even if the young couple is quite poor, these exchanges may reveal to one another their aspirations for a more prosperous future. Instead of political and public health campaigns warning them against the dangers of intergenerational partnerships, HIV-positive women argue that they want greater access to education and employment. They believe that university degrees and steady work will provide them with greater opportunities for relationships with decent men.

As a recipient of PEPFAR funds from the United States, Nigeria has received subsidized antiretroviral therapies and support for its HIV prevention initiatives, among other investments. These projects, however, come with priorities and restrictions that reflect ethnocentric and uncritical assumptions about sexuality, morality, and health. One of these emphases is the "ABC approach" to prevention – Abstinence, Be Faithful, Use Condoms. Unsurprisingly, these programs have been limited in their success. Married women cannot abstain from sex with their husbands and they are often faithful. Married men are much more likely than they are to pursue extramarital affairs and polygamous marriages. Finally, women cannot use condoms if they want to have children.

HIV-positive women are often reluctant to confront their husbands and co-wives about taking a test even when they know they are at risk of infection. If a woman knows her partner's status, she may be unlikely to tell others. She risks being retaliated against or abandoned altogether. A woman has no assurances that her husband will believe or support her, nor will he necessarily seek treatment or pay for their children's health care expenses. In addition to their fears of HIV, women often conceal an array of other violations – not merely their husbands' infidelity but also infertility, abuse, and poverty. Women expose their partners' secrets at great risk to their own well-being.

HIV-positive women confront stigmatizing sentiments circulating in their communities, the popular press, and even occasionally in public health communication campaigns. Their anxieties over stigma temper their motivation to seek testing, disclose their status to others, take medications, and make plans for the future. Nevertheless, HIV-positive women *do* ultimately want to tell others. They struggle with questions of how and when to go about doing this, in addition to persuading others to disclose their status to them.

As women navigate these dilemmas, some will use counselors and other clinicians to mediate their disclosures. Recognizing the challenges women face in telling men their status, these individuals will collude with HIV-positive women to craft a script – whether through a "love letter" or a counseling session – in which men might feel compelled to take a test and then notify their partners. These health care professionals work with clients on their own terms, mindful of what can and cannot be said in relationships. Some of their most influential interventions have come by deviating from formal counseling protocols and instead focusing on the specific needs and constraints that their patients describe to them.

As HIV-positive women's bodies are their primary tool for displaying their respectability and earning an income, antiretroviral therapies are vital. It is not merely enough to be healthy, however. Women want and often need to be attractive. A beautiful appearance may prevent a woman's husband from cheating on her or marrying another wife. It allows her to find new partners and lay the foundation for reconstituting their families. And finally, handsome figures and fashionable clothes are critical for those in sales positions who need to find new customers and earn profits. Nevertheless, in order for women to attend to their bodies with this level of care and effort, they require an outlay of money, which many of them do not possess. Most of the women with whom I worked put the desires of others ahead of their own needs, making it even more difficult for them to save money for their futures.

Women's experiences of well-being (*lafiya*) are intertwined with that of their families and communities. That is, well-being entails the personal *and* the communal, security *and* beauty, taking *and* giving, home *and* work. Because threats to their health extend well beyond HIV, they seek a safety net that could cover all of these anticipated and unanticipated expenses. As women asked, what good are HIV medications and sophisticated laboratories if they fracture an arm in a motorcycle accident and have no money to see a physician? "Magic bullet" approaches involving the provisions of single-targeted medical technologies, such as antiretroviral therapies, are insufficient when illnesses result from a combination of physiological, emotional, social, and spiritual causes.

Of the dozens of unmarried women I interviewed over the past decade, the vast majority desired to marry or remarry and have children. Many of them joined support groups not for the reasons I expected, such as learning more about their illness or participating in awareness activities; rather, they joined these groups and organizations in search of prospective partners and husbands. In fact, support group leaders take an active role in matchmaking. They serve as women's representatives in marriage negotiations among families and even used support group funds to give these couples wedding gifts. Often, the women I knew had no interest in "going public" with their status – either within or outside of their group. A support group-arranged relationship allows them to circumvent the risks that accompany disclosing their status to HIV-negative men. In addition, because HIV-positive couples share the same set of health concerns, marriages may even fortify men's and women's commitment to caring for one another.

Formal and informal matchmaking initiatives have become increasingly popular in support groups and clinics in recent years. The Bauchi State government, for example, made the global news when it reported that it would pay a 40,000 naira (250 USD) monthly allowance to HIV-positive couples who marry. While many HIV-infected women have entered loving and respectable marriages, others have not been so fortunate. Their relationships continue to be fraught with the same tensions and problems that women faced prior to their diagnoses. The social inequalities that exposed women to violence, abuse, and neglect in their first marriages also shape their subsequent relationships.

Antiretroviral therapies, epidemiologists have argued, do more than just protect a person's health; they also decrease the possibility that the virus will spread from an infected to an uninfected partner. Nevertheless, many Nigerians I met disapproved of sero-discordant partnerships, even if couples used condoms or accessed counseling and medications. Most of the HIV-positive women I knew were not only afraid their boyfriends would reject them, they also feared the public's reaction. Elizabeth, who had recently become engaged to an HIV-negative man, cautiously yet deftly navigated these competing concerns. She possessed a substantial amount of information about her illness and her risk of transmitting the virus – perhaps even exceeding that of her counselors. And undoubtedly, Elizabeth drew upon this extensive medical knowledge when she disclosed her status to David. After this disclosure, she took advantage of couples HIV counseling to support her. This only took place, however, when Elizabeth felt confident that he would not abandon her.

Healthy pregnancies provide HIV-positive women additional evidence that the virus will not strip them of their morality, social roles, or the possibility for a long and prosperous life. Children may offer an avenue for securing the material and emotional support of husbands. Men are more likely to take care of their wives, and even attend to their own health, when the well-being of their children is at stake. And, once women have children, they may be better positioned to adopt family planning. Their ability to have a healthy baby, however, hinges on access to antiretroviral therapies, prenatal care, quality delivery services, and skilled support following the birth. Nigeria ranks among the worst countries in the world for maternal and infant mortality rates. One in thirteen women will die in childbirth and one in five children will never reach the age of five. These interventions and resources are sorely needed for all women, not merely HIV-positive ones. Yet, as I have described, HIV-infected women feel the lack of this care particularly acutely.

The Unseen Things has made the point that HIV-positive women share the same hopes and desires as all northern Nigerians – indeed, as people everywhere: to find love, joy, security, social connection, comfort, and well-being. By suppressing the virus's most visible, painful, and often fatal symptoms, antiretroviral therapies ensure that many HIV-positive women's bodies will no longer expose their secret. Nevertheless, the stigma surrounding HIV and those affected by it has remained largely unchanged. Medications alone are not able to alter the overarching social inequalities and material deprivations that prevent HIV-infected patients from realizing these aspirations. Many of these individuals have experienced poverty, violence, neglect, and abandonment – because they lack the social and legal networks to defend their rights as women, wives, and mothers; because they have fallen sick and can no longer provide for their husbands and families; because they cannot have children or because they insisted on having children when their partners do not want them; and, most prominently, because of the ways HIV has fractured their relationships with others. In the face of these threats and abuses, the women in my study committed themselves wholeheartedly to protecting their reputations and rebuilding their social relations.

Kwame Dawes (2008) concluded his poem, *Faith*, about the fears, desires, and lived experiences of HIV-positive persons:

> There is evidence in the body growing fat
> with love, round with hopefulness.
> There is substance in the promises we make
> to protect this world with the truth of our wounds.
> There is evidence in the rituals of the living,
> the memories of the lived, the calm we crave.
> There is substance in the green of rainy season,
> in the harvest of sweet mangoes in November.
> There is evidence in these songs we now sing
> defying that tyranny of this disease in us.

The women with whom I worked often spoke to me with great trepidation but with the conviction that their stories mattered. And, in collecting these narratives and presenting them in this text, I assumed the burden of the "truth of their wounds," as Dawes poignantly summarized. I have tried to do them justice. As HIV-positive women sought to make sense of their lives and convey their struggles to me in ways that I could understand, I endeavored to preserve the singularity of their experiences, the complexity of their thoughts, and the richness of their descriptions. Collectively, these narratives reveal concerns with which women worldwide wrestle as they live in contexts marked by pronounced inequality and endemic poverty. Their contributions to anthropology include questioning the taken-for-granted assumptions about gender roles and family life; the relationships between silence, speech, and power; and the primacy of the body in social experience. And, more broadly, they teach us vital lessons about how women continue to suffer, thrive, and hope for a better life as Nigeria's HIV epidemic presses on through its third decade.

NOTES

INTRODUCTION

1. The names of the persons in this text are pseudonyms. In certain passages, details have been removed or altered to further protect the identities of my informants. Although I spoke Hausa reasonably well by the end of my fieldwork, many of the passages in the chapters that follow have been translated from Hausa to English with the aid of two Hausa-speaking research assistants.

2. UNAIDS, "2013 Global Fact Sheet."

3. See Kanki and Olusoji, "Introduction."

4. Office of the United States Global AIDS Coordinator (OGAC), "US Five-Year Global HIV/AIDS Strategy."

5. World Health Organization (WHO), "Global Update on HIV Treatment 2013." See also UNAIDS, "Nigeria Fact Sheet."

6. For example, see Farmer, *Infections and Inequalities*; Biehl, *Will to Live*; and Nguyen, *Republic of Therapy*.

7. Almost half of all women in Nigeria are married by age eighteen, and more than one-third of currently married women ages fifteen to forty-nine have one or more co-wives. In the northeast and northwest regions of Nigeria, the total fertility rates are 7.2 and 7.3, respectively. See NDHS, "Nigeria 2008 Demographic and Health Survey."

8. Simmel, *The Sociology of Georg Simmel*, 330.

9. Pittin, *Women and Work in Northern Nigeria*.

10. Solivetti, "Family, Marriage and Divorce in a Hausa Community."

11. Schildkrout, "Widows in Hausa Society."

12. See Fortes, "Introduction."

13. For a full review, see Peletz, "Kinship Studies in the Late Twentieth-Century Anthropology."

14. See Berry, *No Condition Is Permanent*, 15. Johnson-Hanks, *Uncertain Honor*, 31–33.

15. See D. J. Smith, "Modern Marriage."

16. Hirsch et al., *The Secret*.

17. See, for example, Tenkorang, "Marriage, Widowhood, Divorce, and HIV Risks"; Holtzman and McLeroy, "Fiction of Fidelity," D. J. Smith, "Modern Marriage"; Sobo, "Choosing Unsafe Sex."

18. Adebayo, "Marital Status and HIV Prevalence in Nigeria."

19. Carolyn Bledsoe and Gilles Pison have argued that a processual and constructionist approach should be taken in the investigation of marriage in sub-Saharan Africa. Marriage, they describe, entails a process constituted by transfers of wealth, the inception of sexual relations, the birth of children, and so on (Bledsoe and Pison, *Nuptiality in Sub-Saharan Africa*). Social identities such as that of "wife" or "mother" are fluid or continually re-created (see Comaroff and Roberts, *Rules and Processes*). Comaroff, for example, formulates Tshidi marriage as a "process of becoming, not a state of being." He reveals how Tshidi try to perpetuate ambiguities in the status of particular relations as long as possible for further use to leverage upward mobility (see Comaroff, *The Meaning of Marriage Payments*, 172).

20. See Hirsch et al., *The Secret*.

21. For example, in 1901, Freud emphasized the ways the human mind systematically censors materials from an individual's consciousness, which may be too embarrassing or painful to recount. He writes, however, "No mortal can keep a secret. If his lips are silent, he chatters with his finger tips; betrayal oozes out of him at every pore" (in Gay, *The Freud Reader*, 215). Psychologists argue that humans often suffer less from the content of traumatic experiences than they do from the effects of keeping these experiences secret – termed the "pathogenic secret" (see Lock and Nguyen, *An Anthropology of Biomedicine*, 285–286). In the psychology literature, see, for example, Kelly, *The Psychology of Secrets*.

22. See Fardon, "Sociability and Secrecy"; Jong, *Masquerades of Modernity*; Piot, "Secrecy, Ambiguity, and the Everyday in Kabre Culture"; and Simmel, *The Sociology of Georg Simmel*.

23. Bellman, *The Language of Secrecy*, 17.

24. Piot, "Secrecy, Ambiguity, and the Everyday," 362.

25. See Ferme, *The Underneath of Things* and, related to the HIV epidemic, Reid and Walker, "Secrecy, Stigma, and HIV/AIDS"; related to gossip and witchcraft accusations, see Butt, "'Lipstick Girls' and 'Fallen Women'" and Stadler, "Rumor, Gossip, and Blame."

26. Acts of "going public," anthropologists have argued, are often viewed as meaningful following cultural logics different from those found in the West. For example, Susan Reynolds Whyte and her colleagues' examination of HIV-positive persons in Uganda portrays the willingness of these individuals to speak out as a virtue that speaks to a deeper theme in how Ugandans deal with misfortune (see Whyte and Whyte, "Treating AIDS"). Similarly, Chris Lyttleton, in his study of HIV support groups in Thailand, suggests that the Buddhist doctrine of achieving a "balanced life" is reflected in public disclosure, as a support group offers a socially condoned way for women to "live [their] life for the benefit of society" (Lyttleton, "Fleeing the Fire," 21). See also Kathryn Rhine, "Support Groups."

27. Herzfeld, "The Performance of Secrecy."

28. Gill Green and Elisa J. Sobo write, "A positive HIV antibody test can shatter a previously crafted sense of self, and it can mean that an individual will incorporate a new facet into his or her identity – that of being HIV positive" (Green and Sobo, *The Endangered Self*, 2).

29. Lock and Nguyen, *An Anthropology of Biomedicine*, 299.

30. See Epstein, *Impure Science*; Nguyen, *Republic of Therapy*; Martin, *Flexible Bodies*; and Rose and Novas, "Biological Citizenship."

31. Nguyen, "Antiretroviral Globalism, Biopolitics and Therapeutic Citizenship," 142.

32. Jean Comaroff, "Beyond Bare Life," 202–203.

33. Das, "Ordinary Ethics."

34. See Fassin, *A Companion to Moral Anthropology*; Fassin and Lézé, *Moral Anthropology*; and Faubion, "From the Ethical to the Themitical (and Back)."

35. Lambek, "Introduction."

36. Das, "Ordinary Ethics," 134.

37. Zigon, "Narratives" and "Moral Breakdown and the Ethical Demand."

38. Austin, *How to Do Things with Words*.

39. See Turner, *The Body and Society*.

40. Adeline Masquelier writes, "Bodily adornments are part of the 'social skin' on which identities and relations are made visible, or conversely, erased" (Masquelier, "Introduction," 5). See also Masquelier, *Women and Islamic Revival in a West African Town*.

41. For example, Saba Mahmood's *Politics of Piety* described how women willfully and steadfastly worked upon their bodies and emotions, through such activities as prayer and veiling, in their efforts to establish a virtuous self. Through these daily practices, their piety becomes habituated. That is, women's outward behavior and their inward disposition merge to forge their pious character.

42. See, for example, Chernoff, *Hustling Is Not Stealing*; Cole, *Sex and Salvation*; Cornwall, "Spending Power"; and Hunter, *Love in the Time of* AIDS.

1. FIRST LOVES

1. For critical and anthropological analyses of these epidemiological trends, public health policies, and gender dynamics in the context of the HIV epidemic, see, for example, Aggleton and Dowsett, "Sex and Youth"; Booth, *Local Women, Global Science*; Campbell, *Letting Them Die*; Hirsch et al., *The Secret*; Hunter, *Love in the Time of* AIDS; Luke, "Confronting the 'Sugar Daddy' Stereotype"; Parker, "Sexuality, Culture, and Power in HIV/AIDS Research"; Setel, *A Plague of Paradoxes* AIDS; and Susser, *AIDS, Sex, and Culture*.

2. For critical perspectives on gender and social change in Hausa-speaking societies in Nigeria and Niger, see Callaway, *Muslim Hausa Women in Nigeria*; Callaway and Creevey, *The Heritage of Islam*; Coles and Mack, *Hausa Women in the Twentieth Century*; Cooper, *Marriage in Maradi*; Gaudio, *Allah Made Us*; Masquelier, *Women and Islamic Revival in a West African Town*; Pierce, "Identity, Performance, and Secrecy"; Pittin, "Houses of Women" and *Women and Work in Northern Nigeria: Transcending Boundaries*; Renne, "Gender Roles and Women's Status"; M. F. Smith, *Baba of Karo*; and Youngstedt, *Surviving with Dignity*. See also Ibrahim Sheme's historical novel that describes the attacks on *gidajen karuwai* and Labo Yari's *Climate of Corruption*, set partially in a Kaduna brothel and in Lagos, where "ordinary" women behave "worse" than prostitutes in Kaduna (Sheme, '*Yar Tsana*).

3. Young men and women, particularly those in urban settings like Kano, are exposed to both global (Hollywood and Bollywood) and local (Nollywood and Kannywood) films, music, and popular literature that broadcast the allure of romantic experiences. See Larkin, "Indian Films and Nigerian Lovers"; Furniss, *Poetry, Prose and Popular Culture in*

Hausa; and Whitsitt, "Islamic-Hausa Feminism and Kano Market Literature" and "Islamic-Hausa Feminism Meets Northern Nigerian Romance." For a specific example of Mr. Lecturer references, see the two different versions of Eedris Abdulkareem's song "Mr. Lecturer." In one, a lecturer pressures a Yoruba woman to have sex, and in the other, a Hausa woman tries to seduce her lecturer.

4. See, for example, Adams and Pigg, *Sex in Development*; Cole, *Sex and Salvation*; Chernoff, *Hustling Is Not Stealing*; Cole and Thomas, *Love in Africa*; Constable, "The Commodification of Intimacy"; Cornwall, "Spending Power"; Hirsch and Wardlow, *Modern Loves*; Hunter, *Love in the Time of AIDS*; and D. J. Smith, "'These Girls Today Na War-O.'"

5. When I returned to Kano in 2006, a new cell phone service arrived in the city, which allowed people on the same network to talk to each other for free. Within that year, everyone I knew had a Starcomms line. Starcomms was different from services and required you to have a second handset (seemingly everyone in Kano owned at least one mobile phone). As this service later began to restrict its free or discounted rates to very late evening and early morning hours, the conversations between boyfriends and girlfriends took on a new layer of secrecy, as couples would speak to each other while the rest of their families slept. Text messages, too, fly back and forth between boyfriends and girlfriends as perhaps one of the most significant ways in which couples communicate. See Archambault, "Cruising through Uncertainty," and D. J. Smith, "Cell Phones, Social Inequality, and Contemporary Culture in Nigeria."

6. These narratives reflect themes widely presented and discussed by women authors in northern Nigerian literature. See, for example, the writings of Balaraba Ramat Yakubu: *Wa Zai Auri Jahila?* [*Who Will Marry an Illiterate Woman?*]; *Alhaki Kuykuyo Ne... Ubangidansa yakan bi* [*Sin Is a Puppy That Follows You Home*]; and *Wane Kare Ne Ba Bare Ba* [*Which Dog Is Not an Outcast?*]. See also Adamu, "Parallel Worlds"; Dabino, *Hausa Love Stories* and *In Da So da K'auna 1 and 2*. For a thorough review of how these works intersect with the politics of concealment and exposure found across Hausa literature, films, and music, see McCain, "The Politics of Exposure."

2. TWICE MARRIED

1. See Coles and Mack, *Hausa Women in the Twentieth Century*; Cooper, *Marriage in Maradi*; Hill, *Rural Hausa*; Onwuejeogwu, "Cult of the Bori Spirit among the Hausa"; M. F. Smith, *Baba of Karo*; M. G. Smith, *The Economy of Hausa Communities of Zaria*; Yeld, "Islam and Social Stratification in Northern Nigeria."

2. National Population Commission (NPC) [Nigeria], "Nigeria Demographic and Health Survey 2008"; Bledsoe and Pison, *Nuptiality in Sub-Saharan Africa*; Parkin and Nyamwaya, *Transformations of African Marriage*.

3. For critical analyses of the ways recent transformations in broader political economy processes shape relationships, see the following edited volumes: Cole and Thomas, *Love in Africa*, and Hirsch and Wardlow, *Modern Loves*.

4. For a review of the anthropological literature on infidelity, see Hirsch et al., *The Secret*; Jankowiak et al., "Managing Infidelity." In Nigeria, see D. J. Smith, "Love and the Risk of HIV."

5. Solivetti, "Family, Marriage and Divorce in a Hausa Community"; the fragility of Hausa families has been a dominant theme in the social science literature for more than fifty years. M. G. Smith, for example, wrote that "divorce occurs on average two to three

times during a woman's life" and that jealousy among co-wives is a common precipitant (M. G. Smith, "Introduction," 26); see also Alidou, *Engaging Modernity*, and Wall, *Hausa Medicine*.

6. Pittin, *Women and Work in Northern Nigeria*; Schildkrout, "Widows in Hausa Society"; compare with Stiles, "'There Is No Stranger to Marriage Here!'"; Keefe, "Women, Work, and (Re)Marriage."

7. Such legal, religious, and cultural violations persist despite efforts by Islamic feminist activists in northern Nigeria advocating for women's rights in marriage. For example, in 1986, Hajiya Aisha Lemu of the Federation of Muslim Women's Associations in Nigeria (FOMWAN) published an article titled, "The Ideal Muslim Husband." Sule and Starratt, in their analysis of Lemu's commentary, note how "she referred to passages of the Qur'an and hadith literature to support a woman's right to go out of the home for valid reasons, to retain custody of her children in case of divorce, to discuss serious issues on an equal footing with her children, to claim a divorce for a host of good reasons, and to expect kind and amusing company from her husband without any threat of physical brutality" (Sule and Starratt, "Islamic Leadership Positions for Women in Contemporary Kano Society," 33).

8. Compare with Hirsch et al., *The Secret*. See also Hirsch et al., "The Inevitability of Infidelity"; Parikh, "The Political Economy of Marriage and HIV"; Phinney, "'Rice Is Essential but Tiresome'"; D. J. Smith, "Modern Marriage"; and Wardlow, "Men's Extramarital Sexuality in Rural Papua New Guinea." See also Renier, "Marital Strategies for Regulating Exposure to HIV"; Schatz, "'Take Your Mat and Go!'"

9. For research on fatherhood in sub-Saharan Africa, see Hollos and Larsen, "Which African Men Promote Smaller Families and Why?"; Morrell, "The Times of Change"; D. J. Smith, "Contradictions in Nigeria's Fertility Transition"; and Townsend, "Cultural Contexts of Father Involvement."

10. Feldman-Savelsberg, "Is Infertility an Unrecognized Public Health and Population Problem?" and also Hollos, "Profiles of Infertility in Southern Nigeria: Women's Voices from Amakiri"; Inhorn, *Quest for Conception*; Inhorn and van Balen, *Infertility around the Globe*; and Kielmann, "Barren Ground."

11. Similar to the findings of Jennifer S. Hirsch and her colleagues (2010) on HIV and marriage, Marcia Inhorn (2003) describes the unjust consequences Egyptian women with infertile husbands face when they hide their infertile partners' secrets, tacitly accepting the blame for their inability to have children. Secrets, therefore, are not only kept to secure social reputations, but they also may be rendered into embodied conditions. Like the Egyptian women in Inhorn's study who protect their husbands' secret by allowing the public to assume it is they who are infertile – actually suffering from infertility on their husbands' behalf – Nigerian women like Jummai both actively and tacitly transform their bodies to establish and protect the reputations of their families and themselves. See also Hirsch et al., *The Secret*; Inhorn, *Local Babies, Global Science*.

12. In her classic text, "Bargaining with Patriarchy" (1988), Deniz Kandiyoti sought to understand how women living within patriarchal systems strategize to secure resources, rights, and responsibilities within their households. While in some cases, she found, women may actively resist these patriarchal structures, in other cases they skillfully negotiate their spheres of autonomy while avoiding overt conflict. And, in still other instances, women will unwaveringly protect – and sometimes stand to gain from – the oppressive androcentric norms and mores within their homes and societies. "Women's

strategies," Kandiyoti wrote, "are always played out in the context of identifiable patriarchal bargains that act as implicit scripts that define, limit, and inflect their market and domestic options" (Kandiyoti, "Bargaining with Patriarchy," 285; see also Sa'ar, "Postcolonial Feminism"). More recently, scholars have raised a number of concerns over Kandiyoti's use of a bargaining model, pointing out its unquestioning dependence on the notion of an autonomous, self-determining subject. Furthermore, it fails to link women's strategic behaviors within the household to the broader processes that set up these rules and the ideologies that reinforce them. Indeed, Kandiyoti revisits her thesis a decade later, arguing that its weakness stems, in part, from positing patriarchy as an entity "'out there', as somehow 'prior' and automatically generative of frameworks within which either acquiescence or contestation could take place" (Kandiyoti, "Rethinking the Patriarchal Bargain," 142). This resistance/subordination dialectic fails to capture the institutional frameworks, historical and political contingencies, and specific social relations that reproduce gendered inequalities.

13. See Abu-Lughod, "A Community of Secrets"; Gaudio, *Allah Made Us*; Kahn, *Self and Secrecy in Early Islam*; and Pierce, "Identity, Performance, and Secrecy."

3. DILEMMAS OF DISCLOSURE

1. See, for example, Austin, "Performative Utterances"; Butler, *Excitable Speech*; Rosaldo, "The Things We Do with Words"; and Searle, "A Classification of Illocutionary Acts."

2. For example, Barbara Johnstone, "The Individual Voice in Language," and Ricoeur, *Oneself as Another*. Johnstone writes that an emphasis on subject positions obligates scholars to incorporate "ideas such as strategy, purpose, rhetorical ethos, agency (and hence responsibility), and choice – without, of course, ignoring the many ways in which individuals' options may be limited or sometimes nonexistent. It means imagining other people not only (or not always) as 'the creatures of their social relationships,' but as their 'orchestrators'" (Cohen, *Self Consciousness*, 93). In short, language makes subjectivity possible. Indirect language and opaque interpersonal interactions – including conversations between researchers and their informants – reveal how ambiguity itself becomes a technique through which humans forge ethical subjectivities. See also Berthomé et al., "Preface," and Han, *Life in Debt*.

3. In his work among *'yan daudu* – men who talk and act like women – in Kano, Rudolf Gaudio (2011) noted the absence of discussion surrounding HIV in this community of pious sexual minorities. Hausa blessings, such as *Allah ya rufe asiri* (May God cover your secrets) reflect Nigerians' deep respect for the Islamic virtue of personal discretion. *'Yan daudu*, argued Gaudio, creatively employ speech, not only to navigate these moral quandaries through the strategic use of silence but also to flexibly situate themselves in both women's and men's social worlds. They use gendered labels, pronouns, styles of laughter, and phonetic practices as linguistic resources to represent themselves as "feminine" (Gaudio, *Allah Made Us*, 199).

4. Das, "The Act of Witnessing." For an example of HIV, see Wood and Lambert, "Coded Talk, Scripted Omissions," and for a broader discussion of silences, trauma, and politics, see Dwyer and Santikarma, "Posttraumatic Politics."

5. Paula Treichler writes, "The epidemic of signification that surrounds AIDS is neither simple nor under control. AIDS exists at a point where many entrenched narratives intersect, each with its own problematic and context in which AIDS acquires meaning"

(Treichler, *How to Have Theory in an Epidemic*, 35). See also Lupton et al., "'Panic Bodies.'"

6. For the second hadith, compare with Nancy Waxler, "Learning to Be a Leper."

7. See also Butt, "'Lipstick Girls' and 'Fallen Women,'" and "Rumor, Gossip and Blame."

8. Leonard and Ellen (2007) label these scenes of disclosure "autobiographical occasions," that is, institutionally orchestrated "tellings" in which HIV-positive narrators are encouraged or mandated to produce narratives about themselves, such as applying for jobs, medical histories, therapy sessions, or court appearances. See Leonard and Ellen, "'The Story of My Life.'"

9. See Nguyen, *The Republic of Therapy*. For a critical discussion of "disclosure ideologies," see Brada, "How to Do Things to Children with Words." See also Robins, "'Long Live Zackie, Long Live'" and "From 'Rights' to 'Ritual.'"

10. Goffman, "Stigma and Social Identity." See also Van Hollen, "HIV/AIDS and the Gendering of Stigma in Tamil Nadu, South India."

11. This observation draws from a broader body of scholarship that focus on narratives as a means through which people clarify, reinforce, or revise what they morally believe and value, as well as generate new meanings, coherence, and mutual understanding in their lives. See Zigon, "Narratives." These speech acts enable individuals to take a stance on a particular set of concerns and thus constitute their identities as moral subjects. See Ricoeur, *Oneself as Another*.

12. Following Laberge and Sankoff, this impersonal pronoun usage "conveys the theme of *generality* – particularly a generally admitted truth or a personal opinion that the speaker hope is shared" and it can be replaced by an indefinite pronoun (Laberge and Sankoff, "Anything You Can Do," 275). Pronoun switches, scholars have argued, are frequently made as a means of identifying membership categories to which the speaker herself is seen to belong. The impersonal "you" may signify a "structural knowledge description" in which a speaker relays "what commonly happens in a situation, so that its use indicates that the speaker's experience embeds them in a wider class of people; that is, that the experience is only incidentally theirs but could be anybody's" (Stirling and Manderson, "About You," 1584). These two criteria are defined and expanded on by Kitagawa and Lehrer, "Impersonal Uses of Personal Pronouns." The Hausa example of /a/ in the parentheses is mine. For a comprehensive overview of the use of impersonal pronouns in Hausa, see Jaggar, *Hausa*. Although the interview was not conducted in Hausa, it is important to note that this was Halima's first language, and thus her switch to the impersonal voice in English also makes sense given how common its use is among Hausa speakers.

13. Erving Goffman draws upon Bateson's use of the term "frame" and states in his seminal text, "I assume that definitions of a situation are built up in accordance with principals of organization which govern events . . . and our subjective involvement in them; frame is the word I use to refer to such of these basic elements as I am able to identify" (Goffman, *Frame Analysis*, 10–11). Frames allow us to make sense of and communicate a particular social reality.

14. John W. Du Bois articulates a theory of stance, outlined in his text, as a public, intersubjective activity in which a speaker and an addressee collaboratively construct and take respective stances around a particular object. "Alignment," Du Bois explains, "can be defined provisionally as the act of calibrating the relationship between two stances, and

by implication between two stancetakers. . . . Speakers show alignment by stance markers like *yes* or *no*, or gestures like a nod or a headshake, or any number of other forms that index some degree of alignment. Just as often, participants allow their alignment to remain implicit, inviting the listener to infer it based on comparing the relevant stances" (Du Bois, "The Stance Triangle," 144). In a later essay, Du Bois (2012) clarifies and argues that "alignment . . . operate[s] as a continuous variable rather than a dichotomy, as participants subtly monitor and modulate the 'stance differential' between them, while often maintaining a strategic ambiguity" (Du Bois and Kärkkäinen, "Taking a Stance on Emotion," 433).

4. INTIMATE ETHICS

1. In the 1990s, global donors and activists sought to mitigate AIDS denialism and promote leadership among HIV-positive persons through a series of GIPA initiatives ("Greater Involvement of People Living with HIV/AIDS"). See Epstein, *Impure Science*; Martin, *Flexible Bodies*; Nguyen, *The Republic of Therapy*; and Rose and Novas, "Biological Citizenship."

2. As anthropologists sought to detail the ways in which global flows of bodies, ideas, money, and commodities intersect with people's everyday lives, they have observed how intimate and personal relations are becoming more explicitly commodified: they are bought or sold; packaged and advertised; fetishized, commercialized, or objectified; consumed; and assigned value and prices (Constable, "The Commodification of Intimacy," 50). In response to these trends, scholars have joined the concepts of "intimacy" and "labor" by emphasizing the array of activities involved in maintaining or manipulating the embodied and sensual needs of other people, both on a daily basis and across generations (e.g., Hochschild, *The Managed Heart*; Glenn, "From Servitude to Service Work"; Bakker, "Social Reproduction and the Constitution of a Gendered Political Economy"; and Boris and Parreñas, "Introduction."

3. Although Binta identified her occupation as an herbalist, other scholars who have written about women "healers" – especially those who participate in cults of spirit possession called *bori* – have remarked on the common perception that these individuals are, in fact, prostitutes (*karuwai*). Adeline Masquelier writes, "Although *bori* devotees commonly assert that the most important thing to have is health (and that is why they are doing *bori*), there are few women who fail to recognize the inherent conflict that exists between *bori* and marriage. Such conflict is often expressed in the saying '*bori daban, aure daban*' ('*bori* is one thing, marriage is another'), which communicates the fundamental incompatibility between devotion to the sprits and devotion to one's husband. Aside from being a potential object of seduction, a woman who does *bori* is more likely to be seen as neglecting her wifely duties and to gain a certain degree of emancipation. Moreover, should such a woman be endowed with special curative powers, she might be able to enough to avoid reliance on a husband for food, clothing, and shelter. This suggests that the whole modus operandi of *bori* challenges the norms of established social orthodoxy in addition to presenting an image of female power that can rarely be reconciled with men's views of the passive and submissive – yet productive – wife" (Masquelier, "Consumption, Prostitution, and Reproduction," 889).

4. Jennifer Johnson-Hanks writes about these competing concerns among young Beti women: "The pecuniary honor of the *yoyettes* (young women) rests on an inherent contradiction related directly to the novelty and ambiguity of women's honor in southern

Cameroon. On the one hand, young women in Yaounde seek to earn their own money and to be financially independent of their husbands and boyfriends in a way that goes beyond the 'separate purses' for which West African marriages have long been famous. Similar to the honor of men, the honor of Beti women rests partially on the sovereignty of a competent, independent individual. On the other hand, husbands and boyfriends should express their emotional commitments in financial ways, buying women clothes, beauty products, and – later on – baby supplies. A Beti woman who is not thus cared for risks losing standing, as would a Bedouin woman who refused marriage and rejected the 'honorable mode of dependence'" (Jennifer Johnson-Hanks, "Women on the Market," 646).

5. Ethnographies of transnationalism document how the experience of intimacy is shaped not only by culture but also material relations – what Scheper-Hughes labels a "political economy of emotions" (Scheper-Hughes, *Death without Weeping*; see also Hirsch and Wardlow, *Modern Loves*). The body serves not only as a site through which individuals articulate expressions of "modern" love or desires, but it also provides the means through which individuals attempt to interject themselves into a more desirable future. In a study of youth in Madagascar, Jennifer Cole describes how these *jeunes* (young persons) will dress "for the futures they imagine." Clothing and the rich array of commodities that women invest in are markers of social status, but they do not merely function to provide immediate pleasure or purpose. Instead, they engender an "anticipatory calculus" employed to transform short-term opportunities into long-term transformations (Cole, *Sex and Salvation*, 110–111; see also Livingston, "Disgust, Bodily Aesthetics, and the Ethic of Being Human in Botswana, Africa").

6. Making a similar observation, Lotte Meinert writes, "An HIV-positive friend recounted how The Aids Support Organization advised their members to 'live positively with the virus.' He explained: 'When the body is already weak you must be careful not to stress it more. You try to avoid problems and worries, make sure you stay well with people and plan for your money and future. Otherwise that stress can get you down.' In other words, he was saying the HIV-positive persons had low bodily capital, in the sense that their immune systems could not counteract sickness well. In this situation economic capital (for buying food and medicine) and social capital (for care and emotional support) were considered important to convert into bodily capital and protect the fragile bodily resources of an HIV-positive person" (Meinert et al., "Test for Life Chances," 114).

7. The idea that bodily practices, in particular, and patterns of consumption material-ize identities and class has been a central tenet of social theory, history, and ethnogra-phy. The "social skin" of humans reveals how the naked body becomes subordinated to social norms and recognized behaviors, thereby reinforcing a shared sense of social order (Turner, *The Body and Society*). In his classic text, Bourdieu (1984) suggests, "'The body is the most indisputable materialization of class taste, which it manifests in several ways (i.e. its shape, its dimensions, the way of treating and caring for it)'" (Bourdieu, *Distinction*, 190).

8. See, for example, Setel, *A Plague of Paradoxes*; Hunter, "The Materiality of Everyday Sex"; D. J. Smith, "Love and the Risk of HIV"; Parikh, "The Political Economy of Marriage and HIV"; and Poulin, "Sex, Money, and Premarital Partnerships in Southern Malawi."

9. As described in previous chapters, Nigerians widely believe that HIV is a disease that transforms its victims into thin, skeleton-like figures. When HIV-infected persons learn that they have tested positive, counselors stress the importance of eating regularly and incorporating nutrient-rich local foods into their diet. In addition, HIV-positive

individuals widely complain that hunger is one of the side effects of antiretroviral therapies (see also Hardon et al., "Hunger, Waiting Time and Transport Costs," and Kalofonos, "All I Eat Is ARVs").

10. Compare with the configurations of competing influences pregnant HIV-positive women face in India in Van Hollen, *Birth in the Age of AIDS*.

5. HOPE

1. Interestingly, there exist numerous earlier Hausa examples of "biosocial" groups such as the *k'ungiyar guragu*, that is, "associations for the lame" (polio victims) and others centered on physical disability (blindness) or disease (leprosy). Renne (2006) explores the history of associations for the lame in Nigeria and suggests an intriguing shift between the colonial and postcolonial era in the ways these organizations structure themselves in relationship to claims-making. Whereas in the 1950s, during the late colonial period, these groups were led by titled chiefs under the patronage of local traditional rulers, during the 1980s (designated "the Decade of the Disabled" by the United Nations), these groups were oriented around taking advantage of state development initiatives that sponsored vocational education and other employment programs for the disabled (Renne, "Polio and Associations for the Disabled in Nigeria"). Cohen (1969) described the institutionalized ways in which begging was supported during the colonial era in Ibadan. In addition to an organization for the lame, there were also those for the blind and for lepers, each led by chiefs who would, for example, collect a certain portion of earnings and take responsibility for assigning the places in the city where members would beg. Among Hausas, Cohen states, begging is a highly organized institution and is based on the Islamic pillar of almsgiving, which requires Muslims to regularly give a part of their income to the needy. Far from being a stigmatized category of persons for their lack of economic productivity, these beggars are granted an important role in the moral economy of blessings (*baraka*) (Cohen, *Custom and Politics in Urban Africa*).

2. Recognizing that stigma and denial produce barriers to treatment, care, and prevention, the 2004 PEPFAR (President's Emergency Plan for AIDS Relief) guidelines stipulated the need to "*promote hope* by highlighting the many important contributions of people living with HIV/AIDS, by providing ARV treatment to those who are medically eligible, and by involving those who are HIV-positive in meaningful roles in all aspects of HIV/AIDS programming" (Office of the United States Global AIDS Coordinator, "The President's Emergency Plan for AIDS Relief," 30, emphasis added). Under the need to support "Social Care," the PEPFAR guidelines list explicitly "community mobilization, leadership development for people living with HIV/AIDS, legal services, linkages to food support and income-generating programs, and other activities to strengthen the health and wellbeing of affected households and communities" (Office of the United States Global AIDS Coordinator, "Care for People Living with HIV/AIDS," 1).

3. Support groups, more broadly, have been at the center of attention by scholars in relation to the effects of reconfigurations of global flows of health information, capital, technologies, and development programmatic aims and ideals, characterizing contemporary "cultures of neoliberalism" (e.g., Comaroff and Comaroff, "Millennial Capitalism"; Collier and Ong, *Global Assemblages*). Rabinow (1992, 1996) has argued that biotechnological developments and the dissemination of biological knowledge, in particular, have influenced (as well have been influenced by) the formation of associational communities whose memberships are based on biomedically and genetically

defined conditions (Rabinow, *Essays on the Anthropology of Reason* and "Artificiality and Enlightenment: From Sociobiology to Biosociality"; see also Ginsburg, *Contested Lives*; Rapp, *Testing Women, Testing the Fetus*; Rapp and Ginsburg, "Enabling Disability"; and Rose and Novas, "Biological Citizenship"). The significance of these biosocial groupings, scholars have suggested, lies particularly in projects involving claims of recognition and inclusion based on a particular illness, or what has been called their "politicized biology" (Petryna, *Life Exposed*; Biehl, "The Activist State"). In the context of HIV, many of these conglomerations investing in the activities of support groups do so to promote claim-making for the rights to universal access to treatment and other needs. Medical anthropologists have described these enactments as *therapeutic* citizenship (Nguyen, "Antiretroviral Globalism, Biopolitics and Therapeutic Citizenship"; Robins, "From 'Rights' to 'Ritual'"; Biehl, *Will to Live*; see also Robins, "'Long Live Zackie, Long Live'"; Levy and Storeng, "Living Positively"). My findings in this chapter reveal not emergent forms of therapeutic citizenship but rather HIV-positive women's desires for recognition and inclusion through enactments of *domestic* citizenship. As described by Das and Addlakha (2001), domestic citizenship is defined by the ways in which claims of membership and belonging are negotiated in the routine domestic affairs of families (Das and Addlakha, "Disability and Domestic Citizenship").

4. This woman's statement alludes to the complicated relationship between stigma, begging, and social activism, differentiating the case of contemporary HIV support groups from other groups with visible disabilities and long histories in northern Nigeria.

5. Smith (2014) writes, "In Nigeria, as a result of lower prevalence, reluctance to test for the virus, and a disinclination on the part of those who know they are HIV-positive to disclose their status, AIDS as a disease is even less visible than in a place like Botswana. I argue that while AIDS the disease remains remarkably well hidden in everyday life, AIDS as a symbol of social crisis dominates public discourse beyond its actual health impact" (D. J. Smith, *AIDS Doesn't Show Its Face*, 9).

6. "Positive Voices" Support Group is a pseudonym for a support group in Kano. I draw from observations I have made and interviews I have conducted with three different support groups of the seven or more groups in this city.

7. Biehl (2013) writes about the significance of anthropologists' returns to their field sites: "Such literal returns enable us to trace the tissues connecting then and now, opening up a critical space for examining what happens in the *meantime*: how destinies have been avoided or passed on, what makes change possible, and what sustains the intractability of intolerable conditions" (Biehl, "Ethnography in the Way of Theory," 580).

8. Although married HIV-positive women must make decisions about condoms under a somewhat different set of risks, it is important to note that most women, regardless of HIV status, struggle with these same social constraints and local moralities surrounding their use. Daniel J. Smith (2003) observed that, in Nigeria, both young men and young women (who were HIV negative or whose status was unknown to them) were more likely to use condoms consistently in relationships that were considered short term, unstable, or based on something other than love; they were less likely to use condoms if they chose partners of good moral character and if their relationships were founded on love (D. J. Smith, "Imagining HIV/AIDS"). Elise Sobo made a similar point among African American women: in pursuit of cultural ideals surrounding, love, trust, and monogamy, which are highlighted in HIV prevention messages, women engage in unsafe (condomless) sex to build and to maintain their denial (that they are, in fact, in risky, unstable relationships)

(Sobo, *Choosing Unsafe Sex*). Furthermore, for married women in Nigeria, Smith argued that the use of a condom is unthinkable: it violates traditional pronatalist norms and would suggest a degree of autonomy that would be extremely threatening to one's husband. It would insinuate that he was unfaithful or, worse, that she has or had extramarital affairs (D. J. Smith, "Promiscuous Girls, Good Wives, and Cheating Husbands"). For all people, risk perceptions and their effects on condom use are imbued with cultural and contingent meanings.

9. World Health Organization, "Guidance on Couples HIV Testing and Counseling."

10. See, for example, Eyawo et al., "HIV Status in Discordant Couples in Sub-Saharan Africa."

BIBLIOGRAPHY

Abu-Lughod, Lila. "A Community of Secrets: The Separate World of Bedouin Women."
   Signs 10, no. 4 (1985): 637–657.
Adams, Vincanne, and Stacy Leigh Pigg, eds. *Sex in Development: Science, Sexuality, and
   Morality in Global Perspective.* Durham, NC: Duke University Press, 2005.
Adamu, Abdalla Uba. "Parallel Worlds: Reflective Womanism in Balaraba Ramat Yaku-
   bu's Ina Son Sa Haka." *JENdA: A Journal of Culture and African Women's Studies* 4, no. 1
   (2003): 1–26.
Aggleton, Peter, and Gary Dowsett. *Sex and Youth: Contextual Factors Affecting Risk for
   HIV/AIDS. A Comparative Analysis of Multi-site Studies in Developing Countries, Part 1:
   Young People and Risk-taking in Sexual Relations.* Geneva, Switzerland: UNAIDS, 1999.
Alidou, Ousseina D. *Engaging Modernity: Muslim Women and the Politics of Agency in Post-
   colonial Niger.* Madison: University of Wisconsin Press, 2005.
Archambault, Julie S. "Cruising through Uncertainty: Cell Phones and the Politics of
   Display and Disguise in Inhambane, Mozambique." *American Ethnologist* 40, no. 1
   (2013): 88–101.
Austin, John L. "Performative Utterances." In *Philosophical Papers*, edited by J.O. Urmson
   and G.J. Warnock, 233–252. Oxford, UK: Oxford University Press, 1961.
———. *How to Do Things with Words.* Oxford: Clarendon Press, 1962.
Bakker, Isabella. "Social Reproduction and the Constitution of a Gendered Political
   Economy." *New Political Economy* 12, no. 4 (2007): 541–556.
Bell, David, and Gill Valentine, eds. *Mapping Desire: Geographies of Sexuality.* London:
   Routledge, 1995.
Bellman, Beryl. *The Language of Secrecy.* New Brunswick, NJ: Rutgers University Press,
   1984.
Berry, Sara S. *No Condition Is Permanent: The Social Dynamics of Agrarian Change in Sub-
   Saharan Africa.* Madison, WI: University of Wisconsin Press, 1993.
Berthomé, François, Julien Bonhomme, and Grégory Delaplace. "Preface: Cultivating
   Uncertainty." *HAU: Journal of Ethnographic Theory* 2, no. 2 (2012): 129–137.
Biehl, João G. "The Activist State: Global Pharmaceuticals, AIDS, and Citizenship in
   Brazil." *Social Text* 22, no. 3 (2004): 105–132.

——. *Will to Live: AIDS Therapies and the Politics of Survival.* Princeton, NJ: Princeton University Press, 2007.

——. "Ethnography in the Way of Theory." *Cultural Anthropology* 28, no. 4 (2013): 573–597.

Bledsoe, Carolyn, and Gilles Pison, eds. *Nuptiality in Sub-Saharan Africa: Contemporary Anthropological and Demographic Perspectives.* New York: Oxford University Press, 1994.

Booth, Karen M. *Local Women, Global Science: Fighting AIDS in Kenya.* Bloomington: Indiana University Press, 2004.

Boris, Eileen, and Rhacel Salazar Parreñas. "Introduction." In *Intimate Labors: Cultures, Technologies, and the Politics of Care*, edited by Eileen Boris, 1–12. Stanford, CA: Stanford University Press, 2010.

Bourdieu, Pierre. *Distinction: A Social Critique of the Judgment of Taste.* Cambridge, MA: Harvard University Press, 1984.

Brada, Betsy Behr. "How to Do Things to Children with Words: Language, Ritual, and Apocalypse in Pediatric HIV Treatment in Botswana." *American Ethnologist* 40, no. 3 (2013): 437–451.

Browne, Kath, Jason Lim, and Gavin Brown, eds. *Geographies of Sexualities: Theory, Practices and Politics.* Surrey, UK: Ashgate, 2009.

Butler, Judith. *Excitable Speech: A Politics of the Performative.* New York: Routledge, 1997.

Butt, Leslie. (2005). "'Lipstick Girls' and 'Fallen Women': AIDS and Conspiratorial Thinking in Papua." *Cultural Anthropology* 20, no. 3 (2005): 412–442.

Callaway, Barbara. *Muslim Hausa Women in Nigeria: Tradition and Change.* Syracuse, NY: Syracuse University Press, 1987.

Callaway, Barbara J., and Lucy E. Creevey. *The Heritage of Islam: Women, Religion, and Politics in West Africa.* Boulder, CO: Lynne Rienner, 1994.

Campbell, Catherine. *Letting Them Die: Why HIV/AIDS Prevention Programmes Fail.* Bloomington: Indiana University Press, 2003.

Chernoff, John M. *Hustling Is Not Stealing: Stories of an African Bar Girl.* Chicago: University of Chicago Press, 2003.

Cohen, Abner. *Custom and Politics in Urban Africa: A Study of Hausa Migrants in Yoruba Towns.* Berkeley: University of California Press, 1969.

Cohen, Anthony. *Self Consciousness: An Alternative Anthropology of Identity.* London: Routledge, 1994.

Cole, Jennifer. *Sex and Salvation: Imagining the Future in Madagascar.* Chicago: University of Chicago Press, 2010.

Cole, Jennifer, and Lynn M. Thomas, eds. *Love in Africa.* Chicago: University of Chicago Press, 2009.

Coles, Catherine, and Beverly B. Mack. *Hausa Women in the Twentieth Century.* Madison: University of Wisconsin Press, 1991.

Collier, S. J., and A. Ong, eds. *Global Assemblages: Technology, Politics, and Ethics as Anthropological Problems.* Malden, MA: Blackwell, 2005.

Comaroff, Jean. "Beyond Bare Life: AIDS, (Bio)Politics, and the Neoliberal Order." *Public Culture* 19, no. 1 (2007): 197–219.

Comaroff, Jean, and John L. Comaroff. "Millennial Capitalism: First Thoughts on a Second Coming." *Public Culture* 12, no. 2 (2000): 291–343.

Comaroff, John. *The Meaning of Marriage Payments.* London: Academic Press, 1980.

Comaroff, John, and S. Roberts. *Rules and Processes*. Chicago: University of Chicago Press, 1981.

Constable, Nicole. "The Commodification of Intimacy: Marriage, Sex, and Reproductive Labor." *Annual Review of Anthropology* 38 (2009): 49–64.

Cooper, Barbara. *Marriage in Maradi: Gender and Culture in a Hausa Society in Niger, 1900–1989*. Portsmouth, NH: Heinemann, 1997.

Cornwall, Andrea. "Spending Power: Love, Money, and the Reconfiguration of Gender Relations in Ado-Odo, Southwestern Nigeria." *American Ethnologist* 29, no. 4 (2002): 963–980.

Dabino, Ado Ahmad Gidan. *In Da So da K'auna 1 and 2*. Kano, Nigeria: Nuruddeen Publication, 1991. Print.

———. *Hausa Love Stories: Origins, Development and Their Impact on the Hausa in Nigeria*. Translated by Joseph McIntyre. From Oral Literature to Video: The Case of Hausa. Edited by Joseph McIntyre and Mechthild Reh. Cologne, Germany: Rudiger Koppe Verlag, 2011.

Das, Veena. "The Act of Witnessing: Violence, Poisonous Knowledge and Subjectivity." In *Violence and Subjectivity*, edited by Veena Das, Arthur Kleinman, Mamphela Ramphele, and Pamela Reynolds, 205–225. Berkeley: University of California Press, 2000.

———. "Ordinary Ethics." In *A Companion to Moral Anthropology*, edited by Didier Fassin, 133–149. Malden, MA: Blackwell, 2014.

Das, Veena, and Renu Addlakha. "Disability and Domestic Citizenship: Voice, Gender, and the Making of the Subject." *Public Culture* 13, no. 3 (2001): 511–532.

Du Bois, John W. "The Stance Triangle." In *Stancetaking in Discourse: Subjectivity, Evaluation, Interaction*, edited by Robert Englebretson, 139–182. Amsterdam: Benjamins, 2007.

Du Bois, John W., and Elise Kärkkäinen. "Taking a Stance on Emotion: Affect, Sequence, and Intersubjectivity in Dialogic Interaction." *Text & Talk* 32, no. 4 (2012): 433–451.

Dwyer, Leslie, and Degung Santikarm. "Posttraumatic Politics: Violence, Memory, and Biomedical Discourse in Bali." In *Understanding Trauma: Integrating Biological, Clinical, and Cultural Perspectives*, edited by Laurence J. Kirmayer, Robert Lemelson, and Marak Barad, 403–432. Cambridge, UK: Cambridge University Press, 2008.

Epstein, Steven. *Impure Science: AIDS, Activism, and the Politics of Knowledge*. Berkeley: University of California Press, 1996.

Eyawo, Oghenowede, Damien de Walque, Nathan Ford, Gloria Gakii, Richard T. Lester, and Edward J. Mills. "HIV Status in Discordant Couples in Sub-Saharan Africa: A Systematic Review and Meta-Analysis." *The Lancet Infectious Diseases* 10, no. 11 (2010): 770–777.

Fardon, Richard. "Sociability and Secrecy: Two Problems of Chamba Knowledge." In *Power and Knowledge: Anthropological Approaches*, edited by Richard Fardon, 127–150. Edinburgh: Scottish Academic Press, 1985.

Farmer, Paul. *Infections and Inequalities: The Modern Plagues*. Berkeley: University of California Press, 1999.

Fassin, Didier, ed. *A Companion to Moral Anthropology*. Malden, MA: John Wiley, 2014.

Fassin, Didier, and Samuel Lézé. *Moral Anthropology*. London: Routledge, 2013.

Faubion, James D. "From the Ethical to the Themitical (and Back): Groundwork for an Anthropology of Ethics." In *Ordinary Ethics: Anthropology, Language, and Action*, edited by Michael Lambek, 84–104. Bronx, NY: Fordham University Press, 2010.

Feldman-Savelsberg, Pamela. "Is Infertility an Unrecognized Public Health and Population Problem? The View from the Cameroon Grasslands." In *Infertility around the Globe: New Thinking on Childlessness, Gender and Reproductive Technologies*, edited by Marcia C. Inhorn and Frank van Balen, 215–232. Berkeley: University of California Press, 2002.

Ferme, Mariane C. *The Underneath of Things: Violence, History, and the Everyday in Sierra Leone*. Berkeley: University of California Press, 2001.

Fortes, Meyer. "Introduction." In *The Developmental Cycle in Domestic Groups*, edited by Jack Goody, 1–15. Cambridge, UK: Cambridge University Press, 1962.

Furniss, Graham. *Poetry, Prose and Popular Culture in Hausa*. Washington, DC: Smithsonian Institution Press, 1996.

Gaudio, Rudolf P. *Allah Made Us: Sexual Outlaws in an Islamic Africa City*. Malden, MA: Wiley-Blackwell, 2011.

Gay, Peter. *The Freud Reader*. London: Norton, 1989.

Ginsburg, Faye D. *Contested Lives: The Abortion Debate in an American Community*. Berkeley: University of California Press, 1989.

Glenn, Evelyn Nakano. "From Servitude to Service Work: Historical Continuities in the Racial Division of Paid Reproductive Labor." *Signs* 18, no. 1 (1992): 1–43.

Goffman, Erving. "Stigma and Social Identity." In *Stigma: Notes on the Management of Spoiled Identity*, 1–40. Englewood Cliffs, NJ: Prentice-Hall, 1963.

———. *Frame Analysis: An Essay on the Organization of Experience*. Cambridge, MA: Harvard University Press, 1974.

Green, Gill, and Elisa Janine Sobo. *The Endangered Self: Managing the Social Risk of HIV*. London: Psychology Press, 2000.

Han, Clara. *Life in Debt: Times of Care and Violence in Neoliberal Chile*. Berkeley: University of California Press, 2012.

Hardon, Anita P., Dorothy Akurut, Christopher Comoro, Cosmas Ekezie, Henry F. Irunde, Trudie Gerrits, Joyce Kglatwane, et al. "Hunger, Waiting Time and Transport Costs: Time to Confront Challenges to ART Adherence in Africa." *AIDS Care* 19, no. 5 (2007): 658–665.

Herzfeld, Michael. "The Performance of Secrecy: Domesticity and Privacy in Public Spaces." *Semiotica* 175, no. 1/4 (2009): 135–162.

Hill, Polly. *Rural Hausa: A Village and a Setting*. New York: Cambridge University Press, 1972.

Hirsch, Jennifer S., and Holly Wardlow, eds. *Modern Loves: The Anthropology of Romantic Courtship & Companionate Marriage*. Ann Arbor: University of Michigan Press, 2006.

Hirsch, Jennifer S., Holly Wardlow, Daniel Jordan Smith, Harriet M. Phinney, Shandi Parikh, and Constance A. Nathanson. *The Secret: Love, Marriage, and HIV*. Nashville, TN: Vanderbilt University Press, 2010.

Hirsch, Jennifer S., Sergio Meneses, Brenda Thompson, Mirka Negroni, Blanca Pelcastre, and Carlos Del Rio. "The Inevitability of Infidelity: Sexual Reputation, Social Geographies, and Marital HIV Risk in Rural Mexico." *American Journal of Public Health* 97, no. 6 (2007): 986–996.

Hochschild, A. R. *The Managed Heart: Commercialization of Human Feeling*. Berkeley: University of California Press, 1983.

Hollos, Marida. "Profiles of Infertility in Southern Nigeria: Women's Voices from Amakiri." *African Journal of Reproductive Health* 7, no. 2 (2003): 46–56.

Hollos, Marida, and Ulla Larsen. "Which African Men Promote Smaller Families and Why? Marital Relations and Fertility in a Pare Community in Northern Tanzania." *Social Science and Medicine* 58, no. 9 (2004): 1733–1749.

Hollos, Marida, Ulla Larsen, Oka Obono, and Bruce Whitehouse. "The Problem of Infertility in High Fertility Populations: Meanings, Consequences and Coping Mechanisms in Two Nigerian Communities." *Social Science and Medicine* 68, no. 11 (2009): 2061–2068.

Hunter, Mark. "The Materiality of Everyday Sex: Thinking Beyond 'Prostitution.'" *African Studies* 61, no. 1 (2002): 99–120.

———. *Love in the Time of AIDS: Inequality, Gender, and Rights in South Africa*. Bloomington: Indiana University Press, 2010.

Inhorn, Marcia C. *Quest for Conception: Gender, Infertility, and Egyptian Medical Traditions*. Philadelphia: University of Pennsylvania Press, 1994.

———. *Local Babies, Global Science: Gender, Religion, and In Vitro Fertilization in Egypt*. New York: Routledge, 2003.

Inhorn, Marcia C., and Frank van Balen, eds. *Infertility around the Globe: New Thinking on Childlessness, Gender and Reproductive Technologies*. Berkeley: University of California Press, 2002.

Jaggar, Philip J. *Hausa*. Philadelphia: John Benjamins, 2001.

Jankowiak, William, M. Diane Nell, and Anne Buckmaster. "Managing Infidelity: A Cross-Cultural Perspective (1)." *Ethnology* 41, no. 1 (2002): 85–101.

Johnson-Hanks, Jennifer. *Uncertain Honor: Modern Motherhood in an African Crisis*. Chicago: University of Chicago Press, 2005.

———. "Women on the Market: Marriage, Consumption, and the Internet in Urban Cameroon." *American Ethnologist* 34, no. 4 (2007): 642–658.

Johnstone, Barbara. "The Individual Voice in Language." *Annual Review of Anthropology* 29, (2000): 405–422.

Jong, Ferdinand de. *Masquerades of Modernity: Power and Secrecy in Casamance, Senegal*. London: Edinburgh University Press for International African Institute, 2007.

Kahn, Ruqayya Yasmine. *Self and Secrecy in Early Islam*. Columbia: University of South Carolina Press, 2008.

Kalofonos, Ippolytos A. "'All I Eat Is ARVs': The Paradox of AIDS Treatment Interventions in Central Mozambique." *Medical Anthropology Quarterly* 24, no. 3 (2010): 363–380.

Kandiyoti, Deniz. "Bargaining with Patriarchy." *Gender and Society* 2, no. 3 (1988): 274–290.

———. "Rethinking the Patriarchal Bargain." In *Feminist Visions of Development*, edited by Cecile Jackson and Ruth Pearson, 135–152. London: Routledge, 1998.

Kanki, Phyllis J., and Adeyi Olusoji. "Introduction." In *AIDS in Nigeria: A Nation on the Threshold*, edited by Adeyi Olusoji, Phyllis J. Kanki, Oluwole Odutolu, and John Idoko. Cambridge, MA: Harvard University Press, 2006.

Keefe, Susi. "Women, Work, and (Re)Marriage: Entrepreneurship among Swahili Women in Coastal Tanzania." In *Objects, Money, and Meaning in Contemporary African Marriage*, Special issue, *Africa Today* (forthcoming).

Kelly, Anita E. *The Psychology of Secrets*. New York: Kluwer Academic/Plenum, 2002.

Kielmann, Karina. "Barren Ground: Contesting Identities of Infertile Women in Pemba, Tanzania." In *Pragmatic Women and Body Politics*, edited by Margaret Lock and Patricia A. Kaufert, 127–163. Cambridge, UK: Cambridge University Press, 1998.

Kitagawa, Chisato, and Adrienne Lehrer. "Impersonal Uses of Personal Pronouns." *Journal of Pragmatics* 14, no. 5 (1990): 739–759.

Laberge, Suzanne, and Gillan Sankoff. "Anything You Can Do." In *Discourse and Syntax*, edited by Talmy Givon, 419–440. New York: Academic Press, 1979.

Lambek, Michael. "Introduction." In *Ordinary Ethics: Anthropology, Language, and Action*, edited by Michael Lambek, 1–39. Bronx, NY: Fordham University Press, 2010.

Larkin, B. "Indian Films and Nigerian Lovers: Media and the Creation of Parallel Modernities." *Africa: Journal of the International African Institute* 67, no. 3 (1997): 406–440.

Leonard, Lori, and Jonathan M. Ellen. "'The Story of My Life': AIDS and 'Autobiographical Occasions.'" *Qualitative Sociology* 31, no. 1 (2007): 37–56.

Levy, Jennifer M., and Katerini T. Storeng. "Living Positively: Narrative Strategies of Women Living with HIV in Cape Town, South Africa." *Anthropology & Medicine* 14, no. 1 (2007): 55–68.

Livingston, Julie. "Disgust, Bodily Aesthetics, and the Ethic of Being Human in Botswana, Africa." *The Journal of the International African Institute* 78, no. 2 (2008): 288–307.

Lock, Margaret, and Vinh-Kim Nguyen. *An Anthropology of Biomedicine*. Malden, MA: Wiley-Blackwell, 2010.

Luke, Nancy. "Confronting the 'Sugar Daddy' Stereotype: Age and Economic Asymmetries and Risky Sexual Behavior in Urban Kenya." *International Family Planning Perspectives* 31, no. 1 (2005): 6–14.

Lupton, Deborah, Sophie McCarthy, and Simon Chapman. "'Panic Bodies': Discourses on Risk and HIV Antibody Testing." *Sociology of Health and Illness* 17, no. 1 (1995): 89–108.

Lyttleton, Chris. "Fleeing the Fire: Transformation and Gendered Belonging in Thai HIV/AIDS Support Groups." *Medical Anthropology* 23, no. 1 (2004): 1–40.

Mahmood, Saba. *Politics of Piety: The Islamic Revival and the Feminist Subject*. Princeton, NJ: Princeton University Press, 2005.

Martin, Emily. *Flexible Bodies: Tracking Immunity in American Culture from the Days of Polio to the Age of AIDS*. Boston: Beacon, 1994.

Masquelier, Adeline. "Consumption, Prostitution, and Reproduction: The Poetics of Sweetness in Bori." *American Ethnologist* 22, no. 4 (1995): 883–906.

——. "Introduction." In *Dirt, Undress, and Difference: Critical Perspectives on the Body's Surface*, edited by Adeline Masquelier, 1–33. Bloomington: Indiana University Press, 2005.

——. *Women and Islamic Revival in a West African Town*. Bloomington: Indiana University Press, 2009.

McCain, Carmen. "The Politics of Exposure: Contested Cosmopolitanisms, Revelation of Secrets, and Intermedial Reflexivity in Hausa Popular Expression." Doctoral Dissertation, University of Wisconsin-Madison, 2015.

Meinert, Lotte, Hanne O. Mogensen, and Jenipher Twebaze. "Test for Life Chances: CD4 Miracles and Obstacles in Uganda." *Anthropology & Medicine* 16, no. 2 (2009): 195–209.

Morrell, Robert. "The Times of Change: Men and Masculinity in South Africa." In *Changing Men in Southern Africa*, edited by Robert Morrell, 3–40. London: Zed Books, 2001.

National Population Commission (NPC) [Nigeria] and ICF Macro. "Nigeria Demographic and Health Survey 2008." Abuja, Nigeria: National Population Commission and ICF Macro, 2009.

NDHS. "Nigeria 2008 Demographic and Health Survey: Key Findings." http://dhsprogram.com/pubs/pdf/SR173/SR173.pdf (accessed May 12, 2014).

Nguyen, Vinh-Kim. "Antiretroviral Globalism, Biopolitics and Therapeutic Citizenship."
    In *Global Assemblages: Technology, Politics, and Ethics as Anthropological Problems*,
    edited by Aihwa Ong and Stephen J. Collier, 124–144. Malden, MA: Blackwell, 2005.
——. *Republic of Therapy: Triage and Sovereignty in West Africa's Time of AIDS*. Durham,
    NC: Duke University Press, 2010.
Office of the United States Global AIDS Coordinator (OGAC). "Care for People Living
    with HIV/AIDS." www.pepfar.gov/documents/organization/84863.pdf (accessed
    November 1, 2008).
——. "The President's Emergency Plan for AIDS Relief: US Five-Year Global HIV/AIDS
    Strategy." 2004. www.state.gov/documents/organization/29831.pdf (accessed Novem-
    ber 1, 2008).
——. "US Five-Year Global HIV/AIDS Strategy." The U.S. President's Emergency Plan
    for AIDS Relief. http://2001-2009.state.gov/s/gac/plan/29761.htm (accessed May 12,
    2014).
Onwuejeogwu, Michael. "Cult of the Bori Spirit among the Hausa." In *Man in Africa*, edited
    by Mary Douglas and Phyllis M. Kaberry, 279–306. London: Tavistock Press, 1969.
Parikh, Shanti A. "The Political Economy of Marriage and HIV: The ABC Approach,
    'Safe' Infidelity, and Managing Moral Risk in Uganda." *American Journal of Public
    Health* 97, no. 7 (2007): 1198–1208.
Parker, Richard G. (2001). "Sexuality, Culture, and Power in HIV/AIDS Research."
    Annual Review of Anthropology 30 (2001): 163–179.
Parkin, David J., and David Nyamwaya, eds. *Transformations of African Marriage*. Man-
    chester, UK: Manchester University Press, 1987.
Peletz, Michael G. "Kinship Studies in the Late Twentieth-Century Anthropology."
    Annual Review of Anthropology 24 (1995): 343–372.
Petryna, Adriana. *Life Exposed: Biological Citizenship after Chernobyl*. Princeton, NJ:
    Princeton University Press, 2002.
Phinney, Harriet M. "'Rice Is Essential but Tiresome; You Should Get Some Noodles':
    Doi Moi and the Political Economy of Men's Extramarital Sexual Relations and Marital
    HIV Risk in Hanoi, Vietnam." *American Journal of Public Health* 98, no. 4 (2008):
    650–660.
Pierce, Steven. "Identity, Performance, and Secrecy: Gendered Life and the 'Modern' in
    Northern Nigeria." *Feminist Studies* 33, no. 3 (2007): 539–565.
Piot, Charles D. "Secrecy, Ambiguity, and the Everyday in Kabre Culture." *American
    Anthropologist* 95, no. 2 (1993): 353–370.
Pittin, Renée I. "Houses of Women: A Focus on Alternative Life-styles in Katsina City."
    In *Female and Male in West Africa*, edited by C. Oppong, 291–303. London: Allen &
    Unwin, 1983.
——. *Women and Work in Northern Nigeria: Transcending Boundaries*. New York: Palgrave
    Macmillan, 2002.
Poulin, Michelle. "Sex, Money, and Premarital Partnerships in Southern Malawi." *Social
    Science & Medicine* 65, no. 11 (2007): 2383–2393.
Rabinow, Paul. "Artificiality and Enlightenment: From Sociobiology to Biosociality." In
    Zone 6: Incorporations, edited by J. Crary and S. Kwinter, 234–252. New York: Bradbury
    Tamblyn and Boorne, 1992.
——. *Essays on the Anthropology of Reason*. Princeton, NJ: Princeton University Press,
    1996.

Rapp, Rayna. *Testing Women, Testing the Fetus: The Social Impact of Amniocentesis in America*. New York: Routledge, 2000.

Rapp, Rayna, and Faye Ginsburg. "Enabling Disability: Rewriting Kinship, Reimagining Citizenship." *Public Culture* 13, no. 3 (2001): 533–556.

Reid, Graeme, and Liz Walker, "Secrecy, Stigma, and HIV/AIDS: An Introduction." *African Journal of AIDS Research* 2, no. 2 (2003): 85–88.

Renier, Georges. "Marital Strategies for Regulating Exposure to HIV." *Demography* 45, no. 2 (2008): 17–38.

Renne, Elisha P. "Gender Roles and Women's Status: What They Mean to Hausa Muslim Women in Northern Nigeria." In *Categories and Contexts: Anthropological and Historical Studies in Critical Demography*, edited by Simon Szreter, Hania Sholkamy, A. Dharmalingam, 276–294. Oxford, UK: Oxford University Press, 2004.

———. "Polio and Associations for the Disabled in Nigeria. " *Journal of the International Institute* 13, no. 2 (2006): 8–9.

Rhine, Kathryn. "Support Groups, Marriage, and the Management of Ambiguity in Northern Nigeria." *Anthropological Quarterly* 82, no. 2 (2009): 369–400.

Ricoeur, Paul. *Oneself as Another*. Chicago: University of Chicago Press, 1992.

Robins, Steven. "'Long Live Zackie, Long Live': AIDS Activism, Science and Citizenship after Apartheid." *Journal of Southern African Studies* 30, no. 3 (2004): 651–672.

———. "From 'Rights' to 'Ritual': AIDS Activism in South Africa." *American Anthropologist* 108, no. 2 (2006): 312–323.

Rosaldo, Michelle Z. "The Things We Do with Words: Illongot Speech Acts and Speech Act Theory in Philosophy." *Language in Society* 11 (1982): 203–237.

Rose, Nikolas, and Carlos Novas. "Biological Citizenship." In *Global Assemblages: Technology, Politics, and Ethics as Anthropological Problems*, edited by Aihwa Ong and Stephen J. Collier, 439–463. Malden, MA: Blackwell, 2005.

Sa'ar, Amalia. "Postcolonial Feminism, the Politics of Identification, and the Liberal Bargain." *Gender and Society* 19, no. 5 (2005): 680–700.

Schatz, Enid. "'Take Your Mat and Go!': Rural Malawian Women's Strategies in the HIV/AIDS Era." *Culture, Health and Sexuality* 7, no. 5 (2005): 479–492.

Scheper-Hughes, Nancy. *Death without Weeping: The Violence of Everyday Life in Brazil*. Berkeley: University of California Press, 1992.

Schildkrout, Enid. "Widows in Hausa Society: Ritual Phase or Social Status?" In *Widows in African Societies: Choices and Constraints*, edited by Betty Potash, 131–152. Stanford, CA: Stanford University Press, 1986.

Searle, John. "A Classification of Illocutionary Acts." *Language in Society* 5 (1976): 1–23.

Setel, Philip. *A Plague of Paradoxes: AIDS, Culture, and Demography in Northern Tanzania*. Chicago: University of Chicago Press, 1999.

Sheme, Ibrahim. *'Yar Tsana*. Kaduna, Nigeria: Informart, 2003.

Simmel, Georg. *The Sociology of Georg Simmel*. Translated and edited by Kurt H. Wolff. New York: Free Press, 1950.

Smith, Daniel J. "'These Girls Today Na War-O': Premarital Sexuality and Modern Identity in Southeastern Nigeria." *Africa Today* 47, no. 3–4 (2000): 98–120.

———. "Imagining HIV/AIDS: Morality and Perceptions of Personal Risk in Nigeria." *Medical Anthropology* 22, no. 4 (2003): 343–372.

———. "Contradictions in Nigeria's Fertility Transition: The Burdens and Benefits of Having People." *Population and Development Review* 30, no. 2 (2004): 221–238.

——. "Cell Phones, Social Inequality, and Contemporary Culture in Nigeria." *Canadian Journal of African Studies* 40, no. 3 (2006): 496–523.

——. "Love and the Risk of HIV: Courtship, Marriage, and Infidelity in Southeastern Nigeria." In *Modern Loves: The Anthropology of Romantic Courtship and Companionate Marriage*, edited by Jennifer S. Hirsch and Holly Wardlow, 137–153. Ann Arbor: University of Michigan Press, 2006.

——. "Modern Marriage, Men's Extramarital Sex, and HIV Risk in Southeastern Nigeria." *American Journal of Public Health* 97, no. 6 (2007): 997–1005.

——. "Promiscuous Girls, Good Wives, and Cheating Husbands: Gender Inequality, Transitions to Marriage, and Infidelity in Southeastern Nigeria." *Anthropological Quarterly* 83, no. 1 (2010): 123–152.

——. *AIDS Doesn't Show Its Face*. Chicago: University of Chicago Press, 2014.

Smith, Mary F. *Baba of Karo: A Woman of the Muslim Hausa*. New Haven, CT: Yale University Press, 1981.

Smith, Michael G. "Introduction." In *Baba of Karo, a Woman of the Muslim Hausa*, edited by Mary F. Smith, 11–34. London: Faber & Faber, 1954.

——. *The Economy of Hausa Communities of Zaria: A Report to the Colonial Social Science Research Council*. London: HM Stationery Office, 1955.

Sobo, Elisa. *Choosing Unsafe Sex: AIDS-Risk Denial among Disadvantaged Women*. Philadelphia: University of Pennsylvania Press, 1995.

Solivetti, Luigi M. "Family, Marriage and Divorce in a Hausa Community: A Sociological Model." *Africa* 64, no. 2 (1994): 252–271.

Stadler, Jonathan. "Rumor, Gossip, and Blame: Implications for HIV/AIDS Prevention in the South African Lowveld." *AIDS Education and Prevention* 15, no. 4 (2003): 357–368.

Stiles, Erin E. "'There Is No Stranger to Marriage Here!' Muslim Women and Divorce in Rural Zanzibar." *Africa: Journal of the International Africa Institute* 75, no. 4 (2005): 582–598.

Stirling, Lesley, and Lenore Manderson. "About You: Empathy, Objectivity and Authority." *Journal of Pragmatics* 43, no. 6 (2011): 1581–1602.

Sule, Balaraba B. M., and Priscilla E. Starratt. "Islamic Leadership Positions for Women in Contemporary Kano Society." In *Hausa Women in the Twentieth Century*, edited by Catherine Coles and Beverly B. Mack, 29–49. Madison: University of Wisconsin Press, 1991.

Susser, Ida. *AIDS, Sex, and Culture: Global Politics and Survival in Southern Africa*. Malden, MA: Wiley-Blackwell, 2011.

Taussig, Michael T. *Defacement: Public Secrecy and the Labor of the Negative*. Stanford, CA: Stanford University Press, 1999.

Tenkorang, Eric Y. "Marriage, Widowhood, Divorce and HIV Risks among Women in Sub-Saharan Africa." *International Health* 6, no. 1 (2014): 46–53.

Townsend, Nicholas. "Cultural Contexts of Father Involvement." In *Handbook of Father Involvement: Multidisciplinary Perspectives*, edited by Catherine S. Tamis-LeMonda and Natasha J. Cabrera, 249–277. Mahwah, NJ: Lawrence Erlbaum, 2002.

Treichler, Paul. *How to Have Theory in an Epidemic: Cultural Chronicles of AIDS*. Durham, NC: Duke University Press, 1999.

Turner, Bryan S. *The Body and Society: Explorations in Social Theory*. New York: Blackwell, 1984.

UNAIDS. "2013 Global Fact Sheet." UNAIDS Global Report 2013. http://www.unaids
    .org/en/resources/campaigns/globalreport2013/factsheet/ (accessed May 12, 2014).
———. "Nigeria Fact Sheet." UNAIDS Global Report 2013. http://www.unaids.org/en
    /regionscountries/countries/nigeria/ (accessed May 12, 2014).
Van Hollen, Cecilia. "HIV/AIDS and the Gendering of Stigma in Tamil Nadu, South
    India." Culture, Medicine, and Psychiatry 34, no. 4 (2010): 633–657.
———. Birth in the Age of AIDS: Women, Reproduction, and HIV/AIDS in India. Stanford,
    CA: Stanford University Press, 2013.
Wall, L. Lewis. Hausa Medicine: Illness and Well-Being in a West African Culture. Durham,
    NC: Duke University Press, 1988.
Wardlow, Holly. "Men's Extramarital Sexuality in Rural Papua New Guinea." American
    Journal of Public Health 97, no. 6 (2007): 1006–1014.
Waxler, Nancy. "Learning to Be a Leper: A Case Study in the Social Construction of Ill-
    ness." In Social Contexts of Health, Illness, and Patient Care, edited by Elliot G. Mishler,
    169–194. Cambridge, UK: Cambridge University Press, 1981.
Whitsitt, Novian. "Islamic-Hausa Feminism and Kano Market Literature: Qur'anic
    Reinterpretation in the Novels of Balaraba Yakubu." Research in African Literatures 33,
    no. 2 (2002): 119–136.
———. "Islamic-Hausa Feminism Meets Northern Nigerian Romance: The Cautious Re-
    bellion of Bilkisu Funtuwa." African Studies Review 46, no. 1 (2003): 137–153.
Whyte, Susan R., and Michael A. Whyte. "Treating AIDS: Dilemmas of Unequal Access
    in Uganda." In Global Pharmaceuticals: Ethics, Markets, Practices, edited by Adriana
    Petryna, Andrew Lakoff, and Arthur Kleinman, 240–262. Durham, NC: Duke University
    Press, 2006.
Wood, Kate, and Helen Lambert. "Coded Talk, Scripted Omissions: The Micro-Politics
    of AIDS Talk in an Affected Community in South Africa." Medical Anthropology Quar-
    terly 22, no. 3 (2008): 213–233.
World Health Organization (WHO). "Global Update on HIV Treatment 2013: Results,
    Impact and Opportunities." WHO Report in partnership with UNICEF and UNAIDS.
    http://apps.who.int/iris/bitstream/10665/85326/1/9789241505734_eng.pdf (accessed
    May 12, 2014). Geneva, Switzerland. 2013.
———. "Guidance on Couples HIV Testing and Counseling – Including Antiretroviral
    Therapy for Treatment and Prevention in Serodiscordant Couples: Recommendations
    for a Public Health Approach." WHO HIV/AIDS Programme. http://apps.who.int
    /iris/bitstream/10665/44646/1/9789241501972_eng.pdf (accessed December 13, 2015).
    Geneva, Switzerland. 2012.
Yakubu, Balaraba Ramat. Alhaki Kwikwiyo. Kano, Nigeria: Ramat General Enterprises,
    1990.
———. Wa Zai Auri Jahila 1. Kano, Nigeria: Ramat General Enterprises, 1990.
———. Wane Kare Ne Ba Bare Ba? Kano, Nigeria: Ramat General Enterprises, 1995.
———. Sin Is a Puppy That Follows You Home. Translated by Aliyu Kamal. Chennai, India:
    Blaft, 2011.
Yeld, E. R. "Islam and Social Stratification in Northern Nigeria." British Journal of Sociology
    11, no. 2 (1960): 112–128.
Youngstedt, Scott M. Surviving with Dignity: Hausa Communities of Niamey, Niger. Lanham,
    MD: Lexington Books, 2013.

Zigon, Jarrett. "Moral Breakdown and the Ethical Demand: A Theoretical Framework for an Anthropology of Moralities." *Anthropological Theory* 7, no. 2 (2007): 131–150.
——. "Narratives." In *A Companion to Moral Anthropology*, edited by Didier Fassin, 204–220. Boston: Wiley-Blackwell, 2014.

INDEX

abandonment: in acceptance of infidelity, 10; diagnosis of HIV in, 78; and disclosure, 162, 164; ease of, 56; frequency of, 8–9; poverty in, 6; by society, 122–23

Abstinence, Be Faithful, Use Condoms (ABC) approach, 161

abuse: concealment of, 56, 57, 89, 162; legal protection from, 67, 69; in marriage, 8–9; and social inequalities, 164

accusations: of immoral sexual behavior, 32, 53, 116; of infidelity, 10, 89; plausible deniability in, 83, 101; of promiscuity, 7, 132; in secrecy, 12

activism, 13–14, 80–81, 160–61

adultery, 96, 119. *See also* extramarital relationships; infidelity

adulthood, 55, 58

advocacy and political change, 151–52

affection: in first love, 45–46; gift giving as, 31, 32; in marriage, 72; in positive living, 151; welcomed, 136

agency, personal, 52, 94–96, 100, 129

Amira, narrative of, 29–30, 43–51

antiretroviral therapies: access to, 18–19; and commodification of HIV, 13–14; in concealment of disease, 155, 162; in hope, 145, 151, 152, 164–65; hunger from, 176–77n9; and nutrition, 175–76n9; in

pregnancy, 141; in prevention, 164; and salvation metaphors, 16; in sero-discordant relationships, 134; success of, 4–5

appearance: as concealment, 3; deceptive, 103–104; in employment, 128; in future aspirations, 162–63; investment in, 113–14; and marriage, 104, 120; in relationships, 114–15; in suspicion of infection, 116. *See also* beauty

Asama'u, narrative of, 38–42, 135–36

attraction: beauty in, 96; gifts in, 31; hygiene in, 128; neatness in, 120

Austin, J. L., 16

authority, 8, 12–13, 58

autonomy, 50, 60, 109, 129, 171–72n12, 177–78n8

Basic Facts on HIV/AIDS, 80

Bauchi State government in matchmaking, 163

beauty: in concealment of HIV status, 110, 114, 155; as deception, 103–104; displays of, 2–3; in fidelity, 110; in future aspirations, 155, 162–63; and gift giving, 32, 40, 51–52; inability of men to resist, 96, 119–20; in income, 118; and normalcy, 6–7; self-care in, 112–13; in social status, 118; well-being in, 118; in work, 108, 110, 128, 157

religion: and disclosure, 102, 130–31, 160; discretion in, 76; forgiveness in, 93; in future aspirations, 158; in helping others, 123; and infidelity, 10; and kinship norms, 9; marriage in, 7; in young love, 30

remarriage: and discretion, 74–76; and HIV risk, 11; and HIV status, 73–74, 132; importance of, 2; love in, 122; support groups in, 163–64; of widows, 56, 61. *See also* marriage

reproduction: aspirations to, 158; as care giving, 120; and power, 9, 55, 58; in sero-discordant couples, 149–50; social, 74

reputation: care work in, 104, 111; ethics in, 16; of families, 74; gossip in, 89; income in, 110–12; infertility in, 59; infidelity in, 56; management of, 92, 104–105; marriage in, 8, 158; and poverty, 6; protecting, 109; secrecy in, 57, 60, 155; sexual, 10, 56, 57

resilience, 150

resistance/subordination binary, 158–59

respectability: antiretroviral therapies in, 155; in attracting husbands, 140; bodies in, 114, 162–63; in control over women's sexuality, 94–95; in future aspirations, 158; gifts symbolizing, 52; and morality, 7; parenthood in, 102; secrecy in, 14, 156; self-care in, 102; shyness as, 34

retaliation, 101, 162

Ricoeur, Paul, 172n2

Rose, narrative of, 112–18

salvation metaphors, 16

Scheper-Hughs, Nancy, 175n5

security, 18, 154

seduction, 36, 41–42, 94–95

seductresses, young women as, 31–32

self-care, 97–98, 102, 112–13, 117–18, 120

self-concept: children in, 128; ethics in, 15, 17; secrecy's effect on, 12; speech establishing, 79; stigmatization in, 13; virtue in, 158

self-sufficiency, 130

sero-discordant relationships, 134–36, 148–50, 152, 164

sex: among youth, 30–31; coerced, 47–51; exchanged for economic support, 98; male agency in, 94–96; as object of exchange, 52; premarital, 94; strategies of university students, 36–38; transactional, 18

sex education, 41

sexuality, 94–95, 96, 101, 161

shame *(kunya)*, 34, 66

Shari'a law, 31, 68–69

silence, 52, 69, 86–87, 100–101, 156–57

Simmel, George, 6–7

Smith, Daniel J., 177–78n8

Sobo, Elise, 177–78n8

social care, 130

social exclusion, 89, 101

social inequality: and abuse, 164; in exchange practices, 18; gifts in, 155; IMF in, 160; and kinship, 9; in lack of support, 165; in relationships, 164; and secrecy, 12; structural violence in, 74. *See also* inequality

social networks, 15, 123–24

social relations: activism endangering, 14; benefits of, 5; bodily adornments in, 17–18, 169n40; deception in, 101; hope in, 153; material resources in, 165; secrecy in, 12, 75; severed by exposure, 157; speech in, 79, 100; well-being in, 118

social resources, 5–6, 104, 125, 130

social status, 6, 52, 55, 118, 127, 175n5

social support, 7–8, 111, 175n6

socioeconomic aspirations, 51, 175n5

speech: as agency, 52; alignment in, 173–74n14; in beauty and character, 120; in cultural context, 16; dignity in, 101–102, 156; and ethics, 81, 100, 102, 156–57; generality in, 173n12; indirect, 83; marginalization in, 99; performativity of, 16, 88–89, 157; and power, 78–79, 88, 157; strategic use of, 100

stance, theory of, 173–74n14

stigmatization: after disclosure, 139–40; in counseling, 13; marriage protecting from, 133, 152, 158; support groups on, 130; threat of, 152; and virtue, 150; of widows, 61

KATHRYN A. RHINE

is a medical anthropologist and associate professor at the University of Kansas. She is the coeditor of *Medical Anthropology in Global Africa,* and her work has appeared in *Anthropological Quarterly, Africa Today,* and *Ethnos.*